AF587352

CANCER ETIOLOGY, DIAGNOSIS AND TREATMENTS

CANCER METASTASIS RESEARCH

PATHOLOGICAL INSIGHT

CANCER ETIOLOGY, DIAGNOSIS AND TREATMENTS

Additional books in this series can be found on Nova's website under the Series tab.

Additional E-books in this series can be found on Nova's website under the E-books tab.

CANCER ETIOLOGY, DIAGNOSIS AND TREATMENTS

CANCER METASTASIS RESEARCH

PATHOLOGICAL INSIGHT

TAKANORI KAWAGUCHI, MD

Division of Human Life Sciences, Fukushima Medical University
School of Nursing, Japan
Department of Pathology, General Aizu Chuo Hospital, Japan

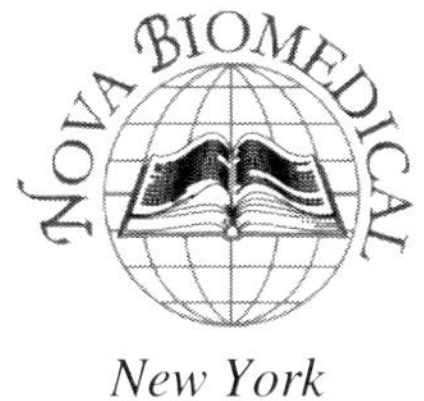

New York

For permission to use material from this book please contact us:
Telephone 631-231-7269; Fax 631-231-8175
Web Site: http://www.novapublishers.com

NOTICE TO THE READER

Additional color graphics may be available in the e-book version of this book.

Library of Congress Cataloging-in-Publication Data

ISBN 978-1-61942-863-8

Published by Nova Science Publishers, Inc. ✝ New York

Dedication

For My Wife Michiko Kawaguchi, MD, PhD

CONTENTS

PREFACE

Many books dealing with cancer metastasis have been published. A large number of these books seem to discuss the topics of the times, and some of them attempted to systematize cancer metastasis. Representative books of the latter type include *"The Spread of Tumour in the Human Body"* by R.A. Willis, a pathologist in England, and *"KREBS METASTASEN"* by H.E. Walther, a radiologist in Switzerland. The former is the first systematic description of cancer metastasis to be written in modern English; its first edition was published in 1938. I own a copy of the third edition from 1973, and this may be the final edition. In the latter, which was published in 1948, the author proposed a scheme of metastatic distribution patterns, which became known as Walther's scheme of cancer metastasis.

My research on cancer metastasis began in 1968, at the 2nd Department of Pathology, Fukushima Medical University College of Medicine (Professor and Chairman, Kyuya Nakamura), and it continued until 2006. From then to the present day, I have been working at the Division of Human Life Sciences, Fukushima Medical University School of Nursing (Professor and Chairman, Takashi Honda) and the Department of Pathology, General Aizu Chuo Hospital (Head, Takanori Kawaguchi). During this period, I have collaborated with many researchers. In 1980, I visited the Department of Tumor Biology, MD Anderson Cancer Center and Tumor Institute in Houston (Professor and Chairman, Garth L. Nicolson), where I studied the metastasis of B16 melanoma variant sublines for a year.

There are three main reasons for my research on cancer metastasis to continue over four decades. The first is with regard to the era characterized by marked advances in biological/medical science. Electron microscopy made possible the observation of the cellular/subcellular behavior of tumor cells in metastasis. The marked progress in molecular biology has enabled the identification of the molecules involved in metastasis. The second reason is the cellular diversity of metastatic tumor cells and host cells. This diversity is extremely important not only in understanding the irregular metastatic behavior of malignant tumor cells but also in elucidating why such populations may display different responses to therapy. The third reason is that there have been advances in research showing that clinical cancer metastasis will eventually be conquered, at least in part. This is evident from the fact that pathologists are now able to report the primary site of a metastatic tumor to clinicians.

Abbreviations and Substitute Words

~	approximately
AH	ascites hepatoma
AMF/R	autocrine motility factor/receptor
BSA	bovine serum albumin
CL-I	type I collagen
CL-IV	type IV collagen
CXCR4	C-X-C chemokine receptor type 4
DBA	Dolichos biflorus
DMSO	dimethyl sulfoxide
EGF/EGFR	epidermal growth factor/ receptor
ECM	extracellular matrix
FBS	fetal bovine serum
FGF/R	fibroblast growth factor/receptor
FN/R	fibronectin/receptor
GAGs	glycosaminoglycans
Gal	galactose
GalNAc	*N*-acetylgalacosamine
gp IIb/IIIa	glycoprotein IIb/IIIa
GS-I-B4	*Griffonia Bandeirea simplicifolia isolectin* B4
GTP	Guanosin triphosphate
HSPGs	heparan sulphate proteoglycans
HGF	hepatocyte growth factor
HER2	human EGFR- related 2
HPA	*Helix pomatia*
HPLC	high performance liquid chromatography
ia	into carotid artery

ic	into left cardiac ventricle
ICAM-1	intercellular adhesion molecule-1
IGF/R	insulin-like growth factor/receptor
IL	interleukin
iv	into tail vein
kDa	kiloDalton
lc	left cardiac ventricle
Le^x	$Lewis^x$
LFA	leukocyte function-associated molecule
LN/R	laminin/receptor
ly factor	tumor cell in lymphatic vessel
m	meter
Mab	monoclonal antibody
Mac	macrophage
MEM	minimum essential medium
mRNA	messenger RNA
MW	molecular weight
NDP	nucleoside diphosphate
PDGF	platelet-derived growth factor
PlGF	placental growth factor
PNA	peanut aggretinin
PG	prostaglandin
PTN	pleiotrophin
s	second
sc	subcutaneous
Ser	serine
SF	scatter factor
SLe^a	sialyl $Lewis^a$
$SLe^{x\text{-}i}$	sialyl $Lewis^{x\text{-}i}$
SLPI	secretory leukocyte protease inhibitor
TGF/R	transforming growth factor/receptor
Thr	threonin
TIMP	tissue inhibitor of metalloproteinase
TNF	tumor necrosis factor
VCAM	vascular cell adhesion molecule
VEGF/R	vascular endothelial growth factor/receptor
v-factor	tumor cell in blood vessel including capillary, vein, and others

VLA-1	very late antigen
VN/R	vitronectin/receptor
VVA	Vicia villosa agglutinin
WHO	World Health Organization

LIST OF FIGURES

LIST OF TABLES

SECTION 1

THE MECHANISMS OF CANCER METASTASIS

SUMMARY AND CONCLUSION

A malignant tumor is a form of neoplasia that acquires autonomic proliferative activity. Three distinct types of neoplasia have been identified: non-invasive and non-metastatic, invasive but non-metastatic, and invasive and metastatic. Non-invasive but metastatic tumor may be likely in a very limited situation, but metastatic tumor cells display invasive behavior in any processes in metastasis. Non-invasive and non-metastatic tumors include benign type tumors such as adenoma and papilloma. Malignant tumor cells multiply at the primary site and then invade neighboring non-neoplastic tissues. Metastasis occurs when these cells are transported through blood vessels, lymphatic vessels, and/or coelomic pathways and implant in distant tissues. Acquisition of anchor-independent growth seems to be a prerequisite feature of metastatic cells. Implantation consists of three cellular events: lodgment, extravasation, and growth.

Three factors affect the development of metastasis: tumor cells, host, and anatomical–mechanical factors. Tumor cell factors include growth factors/growth factor receptors, extracellular matrix degradation enzymes, adhesion molecules, motility factors, cytoplasmic protrusions and others. Some of these factors may be used for autonomic growth but also may be utilized as weapon(s) for attacking the host. Host factors include hormones, immunological status, injured tissues (including the response), and others. These factors may fundamentally be hostile response for tumor cells.

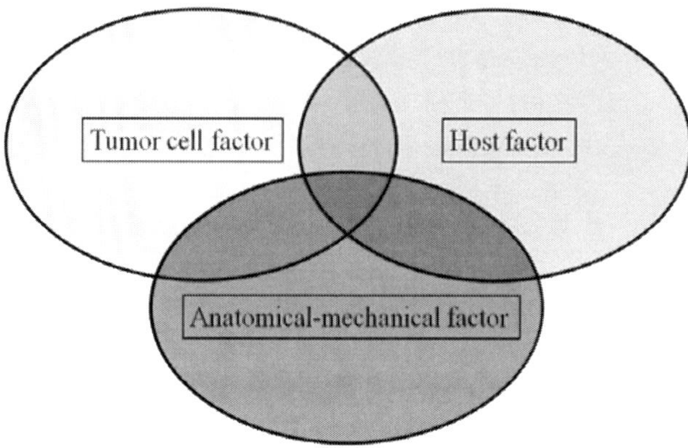

Figure 1. Factors related to metastasis formation.

Anatomical–mechanical factors are basically situated in transport of tumor cells to distant sites, but also, these factors are able to play a role of induction of fertile soil for disseminated tumor cells. Linkage of these three factors induces "metastasis" (Figure 1). We believe that it is important to recognize that tumor metastasis can occur by active and/or passive transfer of tumor cells, and that anatomical–mechanical factor can be replaced, at least in part, by microinjury hypothesis.

INTRODUCTION

Tumors are neoplasm with autonomic growth potential. Generally, it is classified as benign or malignant [1,2]. The criterion is important for the diagnosis and therapy, and cellular and structural atypia, growth pattern (expansive or invasive), growth speed, recurrence, invasion, metastasis, and damages to the host including cachexia are all listed as important factors to distinguish between them. Among them, invasion and metastasis are particularly important phenotypes of malignant tumors in pathology.

We describe definition and classification of tumor metastasis at first and then the mechanisms involved in this process will be followed.

Chapter I

DEFINITION AND CLASSIFICATION OF TUMOR METASTASIS

We define tumor metastasis to be a phenomenon in which tumor cells are transported by blood stream, lymphatic stream or coelomic fluid stream to distant tissues where they proliferate to grow into new tumors. Strict distinction between invasion and metastasis of tumor cells is in some cases difficult, although Willis [3] claimed that "only those growths which are separated from the primary growth and have arisen from detached transported fragments of it are entitled to be called 'metastasis.'" We consider this problem in the following section of "tumor cell transport during metastasis."

1. CLASSIFICATION OF METASTASIS

Tumor metastasis is classified as hematogenous (or blood-borne), lymphogenous (lymphatic), transcoelomic, implantation (aerial), and contact ones.

(1) Hematogenous (blood-borne) metastasis is caused by disseminated tumor cells via blood stream of capillaries or veins (v-factor). Tumor cells in lymphatic vessels and thoracic duct are also drained into venous system. Arteries are rarely involved in ordinary organs, but pulmonary arteries are sometimes involved in tumor cell intravasation. Hematogenous metastasis occurs in general "quickly" and "multiple."

(2) Lymphogenous (lymphatic) metastasis is caused by tumor cells that are borne mainly in lymphatic vessels (ly-factor), transported via lymphatic fluid and makes metastasis usually in the lymph node in

which tumor cells are encountered first (sentinel lymph node). Tumor cells are able to be originated from pleural or abdominal cavities. Venolymphatic communication is also well known [4].

(3) Transcoelomic metastasis is characterized by tumor cells floating in the coelomic fluid, which accumulates in the abdominal, thoracic, pericardial, or cerebrospinal cavities. Transcoelomic metastasis usually occurs in tumors whereby primary sites of tumors are adjacent to these cavities. The peritoneum, mesentry, diaphragm, pleura and meninges are the most common metastatic sites in this type of metastasis. Milky spots in the omentum are frequently involved in these cases. This type of metastasis also spreads further into the lymphatic systems.

(4) Implantation (aerial) metastasis is a type of metastasis where cancer cells are disseminated via cannels upward and/or downward from the primary site to form metastases. Metastasis from carcinomas of the urinary pelvic, the ureter or urinary bladder are examples of this type of metastasis. Similarly, carcinoma of bronchus may cause this type of metastasis.

(5) Contact metastasis. This type of metastasis is described in old books. Lip tumor is probably the best example for such type of metastasis wherein cancer cells metastasize to the opposing lip via contact. We have never experienced this type of metastasis to date.

We would like to describe some terms that have been used sometimes in metastasis. Paradoxical metastasis is a well-known term of metastasis. However, we did not include this in a form of metastasis, because many cases of this type of metastasis can be explained by the routes of tumor cells transported. The atrial septal defect and arterio-venous shunt are some of the well-known routes. We describe lymphatic vessels for the route of tumor cell dissemination, but we do not refer extravascular fluid pathway that was described by Kihara (5). Although this "pathway" has no specific endothelial cells lining it, the interstitial fluid passes through it in a particular direction. Furthermore, extravascular pathways for the fluid flow around lymphatic and venous vessels have no distinct vessel walls. Perineural metastasis had been used, but we do not agree with it. Peripheral nerve fibers are frequently invaded by cancer cells, especially in case of pancreatic and bile duct cancers. The spread of cancer cells in such cases occurs not only by direct invasion but also by hematogenous dissemination. More detailed mechanisms are described in the later sections {Chapter I, Section 1(5)}.

Chapter II

Mechanisms of Tumor Metastasis

Most hematogenous metastasis involves the following sequence of events: (1) invasion of tumor cells into the surrounding tissue, (2) intravasation, (3) transport, (4) lodgement, (5) extravasation, and (6) growth. Similar sequences of events have been observed in other type of metastases. Thus, the metastatic process consists of several cellular events.

Of interest, the term "intravasation" of tumor cells means migration of tumor cells into blood vessels, but it is now more widely used to define migration of tumor cells into lymphatic vessels and serous cavities as well. The same is true for the term "extravasation."

Studies on cellular mechanisms in tumor metastasis have been performed using tumor cells derived from rabbit, mouse, rat, and humans. Microcinematography demonstrated the dynamic movement of tumor cells in the microcirculation system.

These studies were followed by investigations using electron microscopes and radioisotopes. The findings have been verified in vitro as accurately as possible, and the molecular mechanisms in metastasis have been studied for their clinical applications.

1. Invasion of Tumor Cells in Primary Lesion

Invasion of tumor cells at the site of primary lesions is divided into intraepithelial and stromal invasions.

1.1. Intraepithelial Invasion (Carcinoma in Situ)

Primary tumor with intraepithelial invasion is called "carcinoma in situ" or lateral invasion. WHO has classified intraepithelial cancer as the smallest detectable tumor (Tis) and the earliest stage of cancer (Stage 0). This classification is useful when considering the prognosis of patients, but does not indicate the recurrence of cancer. For example, breast cancer sometimes displays widespread intraductal extension and recurrence at the site of the surgical margin. Well-differentiated squamous cell carcinoma of the oral cavity frequently spreads along the mucosa without showing any distinct boundary between normal and cancerous tissue, resulting in recurrence after surgery. Carcinoma in situ of the urinary bladder sometimes shows implantation metastasis without invasion (Figure 2).

Therefore, there is a possibility that tumor cells showing strong lateral invasion have insufficient basement membrane destructive abilities, otherwise they would have been able to penetrate the basement membrane. With regard to lateral invasion, it is also possible that the intercellular connections between tumor cells are too strong to penetrate defects in the basement membrane. Lateral invasion of tumor cells causes cellular destruction of normal counterparts in two ways; one is where cell death is caused by rapidly growing tumor cells, and the other is where cell death is followed by separation of cells from the basement membrane or neighboring cells.

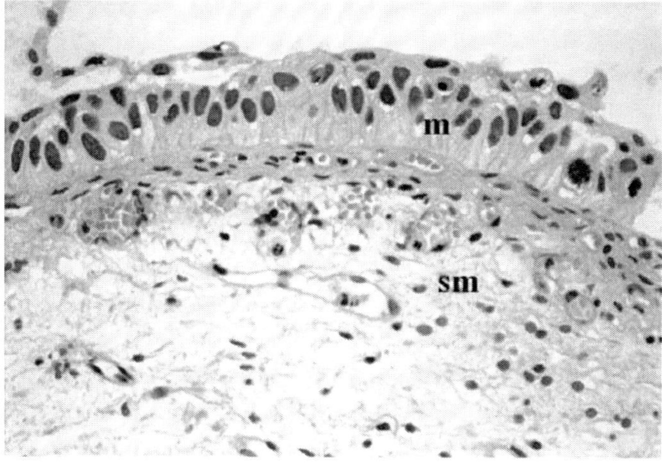

Figure 2. Carcinoma in situ of urinary bladder. Urothelial carcinoma cells invade on mucosal layer of urinary bladder (m), but these cells rarely invade into submucosal connective tissue (sm).

Using electron microscopy, Takubo et al. [6] and Dingemans et al. [7] demonstrated that squamous cell carcinoma cells of the esophagus, uterine cervix, and lung adhere to their normal epithelial counterparts by forming desmosomes and/or tight junctions. Furthermore, they also suggested that tumor cell invasion of normal counterparts occurs after pressure atrophy of the later. This feature differs greatly from that of stromal invasion of tumor cells.

1.2. Stromal Invasion and Invasion Phenotypes of Tumor Cells

Stromal invasion by tumor cells is strongly related to prognosis of cancer patients, and therefore, determination of stromal invasion by tumor cells in biopsy and surgical specimens from cancer patients is important. Considerable efforts have been made to unravel the mechanisms of stromal invasion by tumor cells, and the following three events are considered to be important; the loss of cell junction, loss of basement membrane, and presence of amoeboid movement (Figure 3). These cellular events are considered to play a role not only in the process by which tumor cells in the primary epithelium invade the stroma but also in any invasive metastatic processes. Therefore, these events are considered to be crucial phenotypes of metastatic tumor cells.

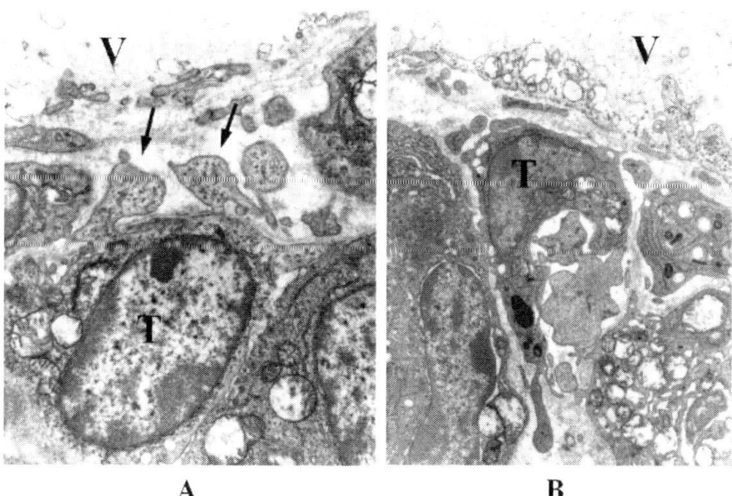

Figure 3. Ultrastructures of early stromal invasion of C3H mouse mammary carcinoma. A: A cancer cell (T) breaches the basal lamina (small arrow) by cytoplasmic protrusions (arrowheads, V: tumor blood vessel. B: A tumor cell (T) migrates into the stroma; the tumor blood vessel (V) is fragmented [8].

A. Loss of Cell Junction

Mutual adhesion of tumor cells in the human body differs markedly among the different cancer types. For example, a well-differentiated adenocarcinoma of the stomach has glandular structures resembling normal ones, whereas a poorly differentiated adenocarcinoma and signet-ring cell carcinoma of the stomach comprise single cells or small cell clusters. Well-differentiated urothelial carcinoma and squamous cell carcinoma are sometimes difficult to distinguish from hyperplasia considering mutual cellular adhesiveness.

Mutual adhesion of tumor cells appears to be irregular, but stable. For example, the differentiation capability of cancer is fundamentally similar in both primary and metastatic lesions, and it is known that the differentiation capacity of tumor cells is similar at recurrence and resection. Rat ascites hepatoma cell lines [9] have maintained their mutually adhesive nature of "free-cell type," "island type," and "mixed type" for over 30 years (Figure 4). We observed that the human gastric cell line MKN47 formed tumor cell clusters when cultured in serum-free medium (Figure 5). However, it is also known that although well-differentiated carcinoma cells dissociate at the tumor periphery, they remain attached at the central region. In addition, the mutual adhesiveness of cancer cells is strongly influenced by necrosis, inflammatory cell infiltration, and infiltration of blood vessels. Therefore, it is likely that the mutual adhesiveness of cancer cells is determined by inherently stable and non-specific factors (Figure 6).

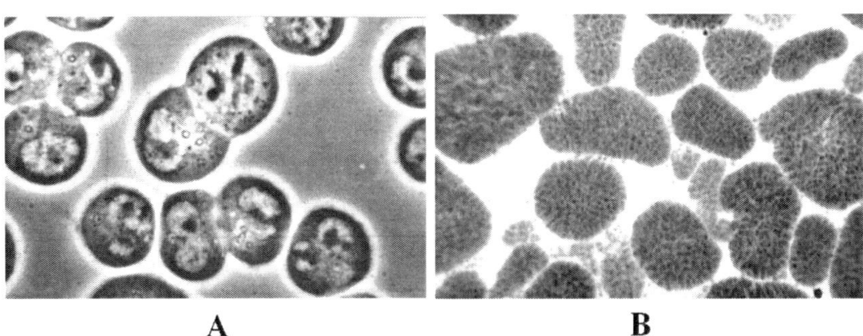

Figure 4. Phase-contrast microscopy of rat ascites hepatoma AH130 (A) and AH44 cells (B). AH130 cells are represented mostly by one or two cells, while AH44 cells form cell clusters consisting of several hundreds of tumor cells called "islands." These images were taken about 30 years ago, and the features seen here can be found even today. We speculate that tumor cells have genetically regulated cellular adhesiveness that consists of adhesiveness and detachment.

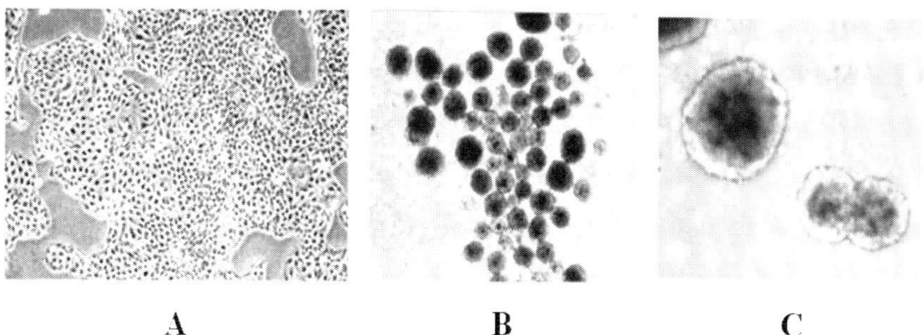

Figure 5. Aggregation in human gastric cancer cell line MKN74. A: When MKN74 cells were cultured in medium containing 10% fetal calf serum, the cells adhered to and grew on the plastic plate. B: In a serum-free medium, these tumor cells floated in clusters of approximately 100 cells. C: Enlargement of cellular clusters. [Watanabe K, unpublished data].

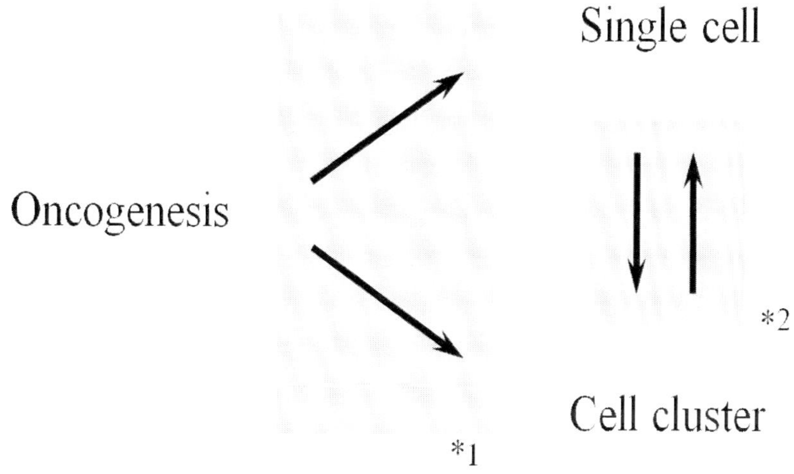

Figure 6. Proposed relationships between oncogenesis and cluster formation of tumor cells. Tumor cells lose normal cell-cell adhesion and cell-substrate adhesion mechanisms in the process of oncogenesis. When tumor cells lose completely cell-cell adhesion mechanisms and cell-substrate adhesion mechanism, tumor cells become single cell and floating cell, respectively. These phenotypes are fundamentally stabilized in every tumor and are considered to be determined during oncogenesis (*1), although they are influenced by internal or external factors (*2).

Coman [10] suggested that the easily detachable property of tumor cells may be inherent, and that tumor cells detach more easily than normal cells by physical force. Moreover, he proposed that this easily detachable property is dependent upon a low concentration of calcium ions in the cell. Although this theory cannot be applied in general, the cadherin family (calcium ion-dependent intercellular adhesion molecules) is known to be at a lower concentration in some tumor cells than in normal cells [11]. Cadherin, together with catenin, plays a role not only in zonula adherence (intermediate junction) but also in desmosomes and simple adhesion.

Therefore, it can be easily understood that the calcium ion-dependent mutual adhesion mechanisms of tumor cells are abnormal, resulting in their easily detachable properties.

The tight junctions of tumor cells, which are a calcium-independent adhesions, are reported to be dissociated by activated neutral proteases [12]. Furthermore, electron microscopy demonstrated that the intercellular junctions of tumor cells were phagocytosed by the tumor cell themselves, resulting in dissociation [12].

Scatter factors, such as hepatocyte growth factor and epidermal growth factor (EGF) are known to enhance cancer cell movement, resulting in downregulation of the cell adhesion molecules in tumor cells [13].

However, these factors appear to be insufficient to explain the mechanisms involved in inherently stable elements such as dissociation of cancer cell clusters at an almost constant number of cells, which is one of the most important characteristic phenotypes of tumor. In addition, it should be noted that the mechanisms involved in mutual adhesion of mesenchymal tumor cells are still unknown.

Apart from the above mechanisms, it is important to discover how the mutual adhesion of tumor cells is associated with their invasive and metastatic properties. I believe that decreased mutual adhesion is strongly related to invasion by tumor cells because cancer cells with lesser mutual adhesion mechanisms move more easily than those with more. We observed that tumor cells separated from poorly differentiated carcinomas invaded surrounding tissues more aggressively than those forming clusters from well-differentiated carcinomas.

Metastasis, on the other hand, appears to occur not only in tumor cells with poor mutual adhesion but also in those with well-differentiated clusters. For example, a poorly differentiated adenocarcinoma of the stomach metastasizes to the lymph nodes, whereas a well-differentiated adenocarcinoma metastasizes to the liver. Island-forming cells of rat ascites hepatoma metastasize to the brain parenchyma, but not to the brain meninges. In contrast, free cells of rat ascites hepatoma metastasize to the brain meninges but not to the brain parenchyma. That brain parenchyma metastasis by these cell lines is related strongly with cluster of cancer cells will be shown later [14]. Therefore, it is suggested that the mutual adhesiveness of tumor cells is one of the causes of diversity in tumor metastasis.

B. Loss of Basement Membrane

Electron microscopy and immunohistochemical studies began in the 1960s and 1980s, respectively, to elucidate the cellular and molecular mechanisms of tumor invasion and metastasis.

These studies frequently demonstrated the discontinuous and/or double-layered basement membrane of tumor cells, although it appears normal under conventional light microscopy. In general, it could be considered that dissociated cells constituting poorly differentiated carcinomas have an insufficient or no basement membrane, whereas well-differentiated tumor cells have a continuous, but not complete, basement membrane [15, 16]. Loss of basement membrane of malignant tumor cells is considered to be due to the following two ways.

B.1. Degradation of Basement Membrane

In this event, tumor cells degrade their own basement membrane or other basement membranes that they encounter during the processes of invasion and metastasis.

Since the pioneering studies by Liotta et al. [17] and Nakajima et al. [18], many studies have been performed on the degradation of the basement membrane by tumor cells and, in summary, the results suggests that metalloproteinase, serine protease, cysteine protease, and endoglycosidase were all involved in this process.

The major component of the basement membrane is type IV collagen (CL-IV), whereas, laminin (LN), fibronectin (FN), heparan sulfate proteoglycan (HSPGs), and entactin are relatively minor components. Similar to the observations by several investigators, we found considerably higher levels of proteases in poorly differentiated as opposed to well-differentiated gastric adenocarcinoma cells (Figure 7) [19].

However, it should be noted that the capability of tumor cells to destroy extracellular matrix (ECM) including the basement membrane (BM), can be estimated by zymography assay on a concentrated culture medium. The degradation of the basement membrane by tumor cells in vivo is localized at the tips of the cytoplasmic processes, as demonstrated ultrastructurally by us [20, 21] and Liotta [22] who proposed a three-step hypothesis for the degradation of the BM by tumor cells.

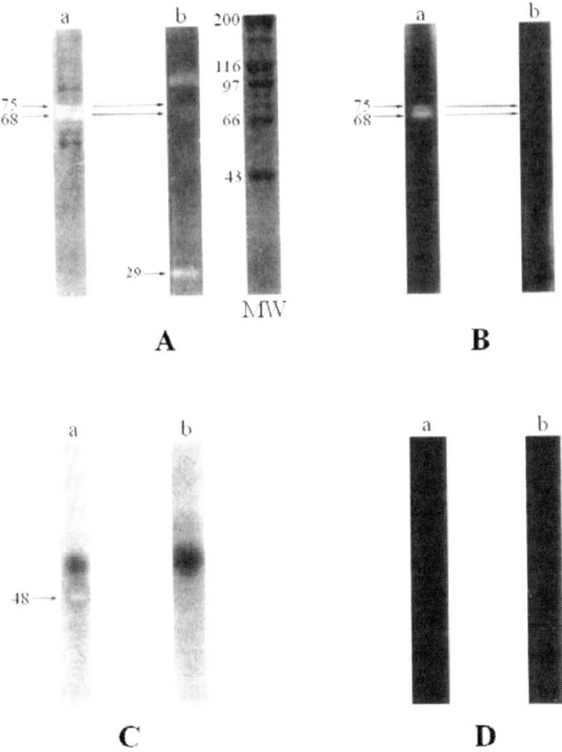

Figure 7. Degradation of extracellular matrix (ECM) components detected by zymogram. Lanes "a" and "b" are serum-free culture media from MKN 45 (derived from well-differentiated adenocarcinoma of stomach) and MKN 28 (derived from poorly differentiated adenocarcinoma of stomach), respectively. The substrates examined are fibronectin (FN) (A), gelatin (B), type I collagen (CL-1) (C), and type IV collagen (D). Two zones (approximate molecular weight (MW) 75 and 68 kDa) of FN lysis and gelatin lysis are clearly seen in the lanes of the MKN 45 medium (A-a, B-a) but weaker in the MKN 28 medium (A-b, B-b). ~29 kDa FN lysis and 100–150 kDa FN and gelatinolysis were detected in the MKN 28 medium (A-b, B-b). Type I collagen-degrading activity of 48 kDa was detected only in the MKN 45 medium (C-a). Type IV collagen degradation was not observed in either tumor line (D, a, b) [19].

B.2. Insufficient Ability to Produce Basement Membrane Component Including Irregular Polarity

There are several factors that may lead to this insufficiency. Invasive ductal carcinoma cells of the breast rarely form a basement membrane, as these cells do not possess myoepithelial cell characteristics. Another possibility is that tumor cells produce BM components but cannot constitute the BM itself.

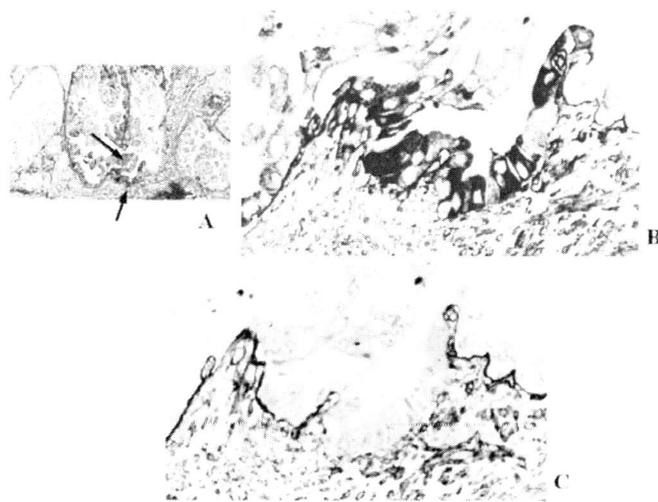

Figure 8. Laminin and type IV collagen expression in human gastric cancer. A: Anti-LN antibody stain. Large areas of the basement membrane are stained with anti-LN antibody. B: Enlargement of the area is indicated by arrowheads in A. Cancer cell cytoplasm was stained with anti-LN antibody, but corresponding areas of the BM were not stained. C: Anti-CL-IV staining of the same area as shown in B. [Kawaguchi T, unpublished data].

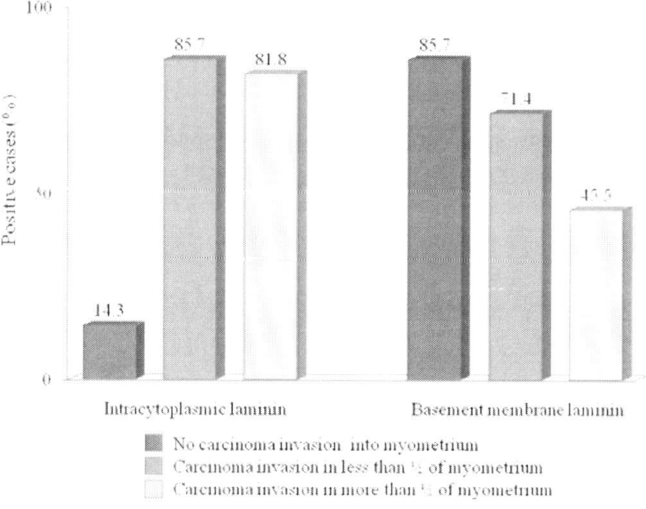

Figure 9. Positive laminin staining of human endometrial cancer cells according to myometrial invasion. The level of LN in cancer cells and/or basement membrane appears to be related to myometrial invasion by cancer cells [23].

For example, we found that cells of human gastric cancer, a type of papillotubular carcinoma, have their BM almost completely surrounding the gland, but they lack the BM components LN and type IV in those areas where LN appears in the cancer cells (Figure 8). In human endometrial cancer (endometrioid adenocarcinoma), we found a positive relationship between LN deposits in cancer cell cytoplasm and the depth of myometrial invasion, and a negative relationship between the presence of LN in the basement membrane and the depth of invasion (Figure 9) [23]. Irregular transport of ECM, CL-IV, and LN is involved in these cases.

C. Locomotion

Similar to non-tumorous cells, locomotion of tumor cells are a complex phenomenon, which is governed by locomotion signals and occurs as a sequence of events such as adhesion to normal cells and/or stroma, movement, and detachment. It is a well-known fact that certain molecules derived from tumor tissues, serum, and complements are all able to promote tumor cell locomotion, and recently these molecular mechanisms have been studied in detail. In addition, recent studies have demonstrated that tumor cells secrete a motility factor including autocrine motility factor, while other tissues express a tumor invasion-inhibiting factor. Although numerous factors/molecules have been reported to be involved, there are no reliable motility factor(s) specific for cancer cells. It is especially important to identify the molecular mechanisms that mediate intravasation and extravasation by tumor cells. The locomotion factors involved in every metastatic process will be described in the latter section, and fundamental aspects of locomotion by invasive tumor cells will also be described. Here, we would like to emphasize that tumor cell movement is achieved by not only tumor cells themselves but also by host cells such as vascular endothelial cells and stromal cells. The latter makes us propose a new concept of invasion and metastasis.

Invasion of tumor cells into interstitial tissue (stromal invasion) is strongly influenced by the tissues that tumor cells encounter. Cartilage, artery, valve, cornea, and vitreous body appear to be resistant for tumor cell invasion. Resistance of cartilaginous tissue by tumor cell invasion is well-known fact. For example, osteosarcoma cells invade destructively into bone marrow and bone cortex, but these cells rarely invade into epiphyseal cartilage. And even though invasion is seen, it occurs along blood vessels. The resistance of cartilage against tumor invasion may be explained by their peculiar arrangement of cartilagenous fibers and/or protease inhibitors [24]. Less resistance against tumor invasion is seen in loose connective tissues where lymphatic vessels and extravascular fluid pathways exist, and actually, any kinds of tumor cells spread in this tissues. Therefore, it is natural to consider that mechanical barrier is involved in resistance against tumor invasion.

On the other hand, it is apparent that some kinds of tumor cells invade strongly into muscle tissues, nerve tissues, and venous tissues, which are all dense connective tissues. These tissues are characterized by the presence of abundant BM components, which contain much CL-IV, LN, HSPGs, and FN, and these ECMs are possible to provide fertile soil for cancer cell migration [25].

Like normal tissues, tumor cells invade in pathological tissues of necrotic tissues and granulation tissues, although these cells tend to avoid scar tissues. Especially, tumor cells prefer to grow in granulation tissues. It is a well-known fact that granulation tissues contain various kinds of growth factors, cytokines, and proteases in large amounts, as reported by Sylven in 1967 [26]. More recently, it was demonstrated that granulation tissues contained TGF-β, bFGF and HGF, these growth factors having strong induction abilities to fibroblasts, myofibroblasts and blood vessels as well as chemotactic activities [27]. It is also reported that tumor tissues involve peculiar extracellular matrices like tenascin and oncofetal fibronectin. Tenascin appears to promote liberation of cancer cells from substrates [28].

1.3. Mechanisms of Destructive Action of Tumor Cells on Host Cells

Pathologists have occasionally observed that invasive growth of tumor cells accompanied tissue injuries of host. This includes destruction of stromal tissues as well as parenchymal ones, possibly resulting from the pressure caused by the expansive growth of tumor cells, invasive growth of tumor cells, and/or proteolytic enzymes including toxohormone [29]. We would like to describe a very interesting phenomenon, indicating that tumor cells destroy tissue parenchymal cells by their direct action. This phenomenon is considered to be very important because it appears to be one of the features of the malignant phenotype of tumor cells, although no systemic studies to validate this have been conducted so far.

Ultrastructural studies on the mechanisms involved in destructive invasion of skeletal and smooth muscles by L 1210 leukemia cells were performed in the 1960s, by Brandes [30], followed by Galasko et al. [31] and Gabbert et al. [32].

We have conducted an ultrastructural study on the invasion of a primary cultured adult rat hepatocyte monolayer by rat ascites hepatoma variant sublines (74AD, 74FL) (Figure 10, 11) [33]. Although 74AD and 74FL are an adherent and a floating sublines, respectively, in ordinary in vivo culture (see Chapter III, Section 2), most of the cells of both sublines attached to the hepatocytes at the tips of their cytoplasmic processes for up to two hours after co-culture. Thereafter, these cells adhered to the hepatocytes with several types of junctional structures. Simple apposition was prominent six hours after co-culture, and intermediate and tight junctions were frequently observed after 12 hours. The attached tumor cells separated the intercellular junctions of the hepatocyte monolayer with their cytoplasmic protrusions and directly adhered to the dish by pushing aside the hepatocytes. In addition, after 12 hours of co-culture, we sometimes found a peculiar interaction that appeared to be an early event in cytoplasmic fusion between a tumor cell and a hepatocyte. Increased electron density of mitochondria, disappearance of cristae, and presence of cytoplasmic vacuolations were observed in the hepatocytes fused with tumor cells. These observations suggest that the hepatic invasion by tumor cells results from an interaction between tumor cells and hepatocytes leading to their cytoplasmic fusion, as well as direct migration of tumor cells into hepatic cords. The mechanism of invasion may be independent of substrate adhesion.

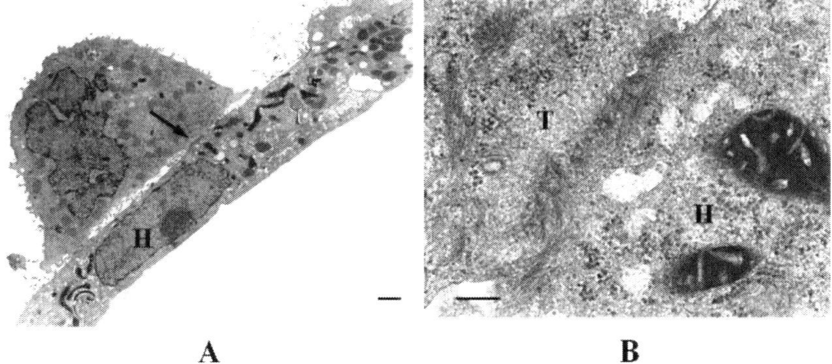

Figure 10. Partial cytoplasmic cell fusion between a 74AD cell and a hepatocyte after 48 hour of co-culture. A: A 74AD cell (A) adheres to a hepatocyte (H) at several sites. At this low magnification, one of them appears to be a tight junction. Bar = 2 μm. B: Higher magnification of the arrow site (↑). Numerous microtubules mingle in the tumor cell (T) – hepatocyte (H) boundary, and no distinct cellular boundary between the two cells was found in this area. Bar = 200 nm [33].

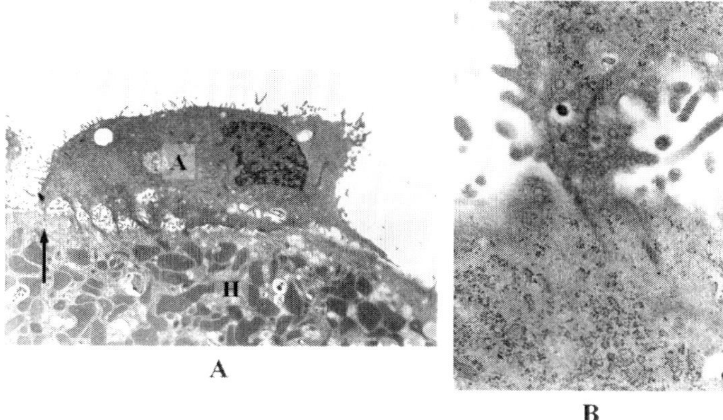

Figure 11. A peculiar interaction between 74FL cell and a hepatocyte after 12 h co-culture. A: 74FL cells appear to insert their slender cytoplasmic protrusions into the hepatocyte. The hepatocytes display slight degenerative changes, such as an increase in the electron density of mitochondria, disappearance of the mitochondria cristiae, and cytoplasmic vacuolations. A = 74FL; H = hepatocyte. Bar = 2μ. B: A higher magnification of the area at an arrow. The cytoplasmic projection contains microtubules [33].

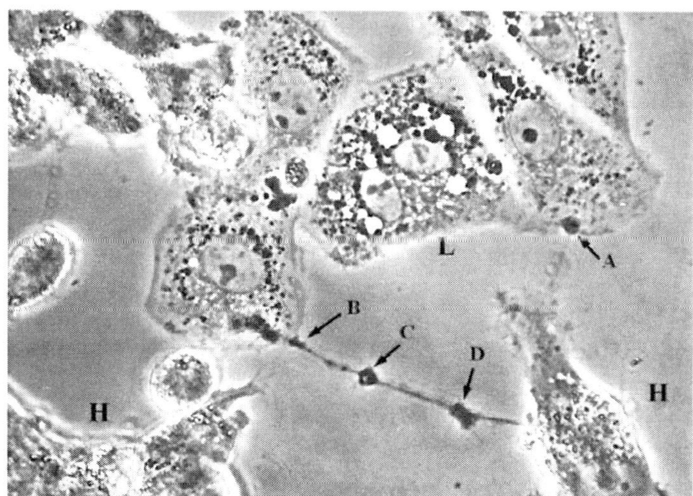

Figure 12. Phase contrast photomicrograph of a mixed culture of normal liver cells of strain RCL-1 (L) and ascites hepatoma AH130 cells (H) of rat. Hepatoma cells are adhering to liver cells at A and B. Small swellings (C and D) in the cytoplasmic projections of the hepatoma cells are due to materials absorbed by pinocytosis or phagocytosis from liver cells and are being transported towards the cytoplasm of hepatoma cells [34] (with permissions of author and publisher).

Apart from our studies, Katsuta et al. [34] studied the interaction between tumor and normal cells in vitro. They observed by cinematomicrography the behavior of rat ascites hepatoma AH130 cells mixed with normal rat liver cells of the strain RCL-1. The results were striking. The hepatoma cells approached the normal liver cells and actively attached themselves to the liver cells by cell contact. They stretched out their cytoplasmic protrusions toward the liver cells and adhered to their cytoplasm, using the tips of protrusions like suckers. They appeared to absorb the nutritional substances present in the cytoplasm of liver cells through these suckers, by pinocytosis and phagocytosis, and/or to inject toxic metabolites in the liver cells (Figure 12). The liver cells gradually underwent pyknosis, and the movement of cytoplasmic granules was noticeably suppressed. Within a week in this mixed culture, the liver cells diminished in population, probably having been phagocytosed by the hepatoma cells.

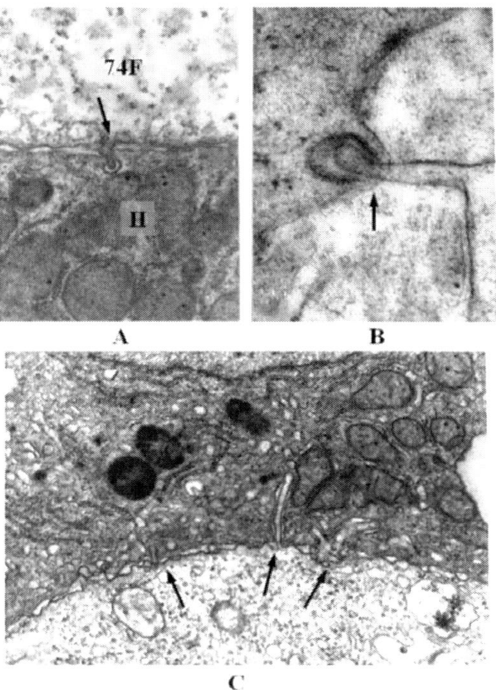

Figure 13. Attack of rat ascites hepatoma AH7974F (74F) against a hepatocyte (H) in rat. Invagination of a cytoplasmic protrusion of a tumor cell into a coated vesicle in a hepatic cell (arrow). A: 12 hours after intravenous (i.v.) injection. B: Four days after i.v. injection. C: Cytoplasmic protrusion of a tumor cell invaginated in the coated vesicles and intruded into the hepatic cells. Four days after i.v. injection [21].

We noted a similar destruction pattern of the hepatocytes, nerve cells, and endothelial cells by cancer cells in vivo [21, 35-37]. We surmise that a particular tumor cell type is able to attach to normal cells in a tight junction-like manner, followed by insertion of cytoplasmic protrusions, resulting in destruction of host cells (Figure 13).

1.4. Enclosure and Engulfment of Tumor Cells by Host Mesenchymal Cells

We have reported that tumor cells are enclosed by host cells mostly by endothelial cells, mesothelial cells, or myofibroblasts (see next section). We first noticed such interactions when the lodgement and extravasation of tumor cells in the brain were examined by electron microscopy. In this case, tumor cells were enclosed by endothelial cells of cerebral capillaries. No basement membrane intervened between the tumor and endothelial cells, indicating that the tumor cells were attached to the endothelial cells. We also observed a similar interaction when tumor cells were arrested in the sinusoidal blood vessels of the liver.

A striking observation was that Yoshida sarcoma cells were enclosed by the endothelial cells of lymphatic vessels. Please refer to the section on intravasation of tumor cells (Figure 18). Such an interaction was frequently observed between Yoshida sarcoma cells and repaired mesothelial cells of the abdominal wall [38]. Therefore, we consider that the interaction between tumor and host mesenchymal cells, such as the endothelial cells of blood vessels and lymphatic vessels and mesothelial cells, plays an important role in the development of tumor metastasis.

Another important observation was the interaction between tumor cells and myofibroblasts (Figure 14). We first noticed this interaction during electron microscopic examinations of gastric cancer cell invasion. In this case, cancer cells appear to be enclosed by filamentous cytoplasmic protrusions of myofibroblasts. In some cases, we could not distinguish these cytoplasmic protrusions from those of the endothelial cells of lymphatic vessels. Similar findings were observed in the human invasive ductal carcinoma of the pancreas, in which cancer cells were enclosed by myofibroblasts. We have not studied this interaction in detail in terms of its mechanisms and roles in invasion. We speculate this interaction being advantageous for the unchecked growth of tumor cells because we never observed destroyed tumor cells among them.

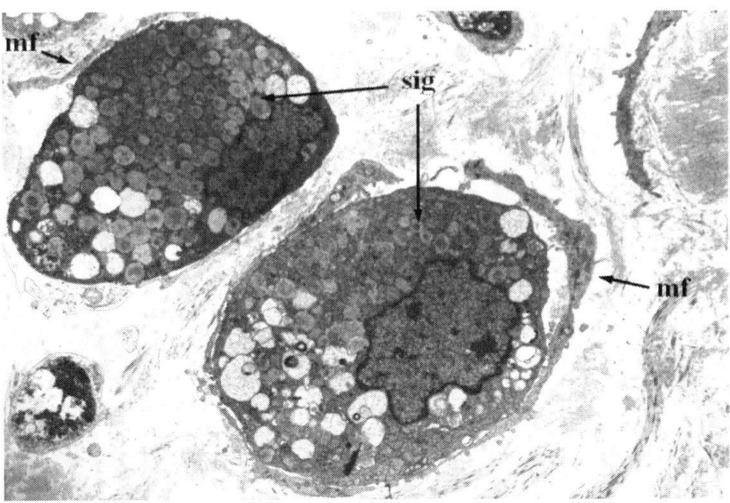

Figure 14. Interaction of a cancer cell and a myofibroblast. Signet-ring cell carcinoma cells (sig) of stomach are enclosed by cytoplasmic protrusions of myofibroblasts (mf) [Kawaguchi T, unpublished data].

Direct interaction between tumor and hematopoietic cells, including inflammatory cells such as neutrophils, seems to occur frequently. Although we could not obtain any valuable information regarding the interaction between tumor and hematopoietic cells, some researchers have claimed that this interaction might be associated with tumor progression [39]. We aim to collate more information on the same in a future study. Apart from direct interactions, various kinds of interactions that are related to tumor invasion and metastasis exist between tumor cells and host tissues. These include induction of tumor blood vessels (tumor angiogenesis) and depression of tumor-specific immunity.

1.5. Commentary: Nerve Invasion

The spread of tumor via peripheral nerve fibers is considered important because the invasion of peripheral nerve fiber (pn/neu-factor) is a prognostic factor in the diagnosis of pancreatic, bile duct, and prostatic cancers [40, 41]. There are two evident routes of peripheral nerve fiber invasion: direct invasion and via hematogenous dissemination. Here, we refer to the perineural spread of malignant tumors. Since the early part of last century, it has been generally believed that tumor growth takes place within the spaces or lymphatic channels of peripheral nerves.

However, transmission electron microscopy did not reveal any spaces and/or lymphatic channels, suggesting that the supposed perineural spaces represent areas of least resistance to tumor invasion.

Animal studies using dye injections have shown that prostatic lymphatics are distributed around prostatic ducts and are in close relation with blood capillaries; however, prostatic lymphatic vessels showed no relationship to nerves.

It was also demonstrated that injection of tumor cells into the perineurium of peripheral nerves in rats led to tumor cell growth within the nerve or in the perineural sheath but not within lymphatic vessels [42]. Therefore, we consider that perineural and neural involvement of tumor is not related to metastasis but invasion.

2. Intravasation: Migration of Tumor Cells into Blood Vessels, Lymphatic Vessels, and Coelomic Cavities

Metastasis begins when tumor cells enter blood vessels, lymphatic vessels, or coelomic cavities. Intravasation is one of the determinants of tumor metastasis, as numerous investigators have reported a positive correlation between vascular involvement (v-factor) and metastasis/prognosis in patients with various types of malignant tumors. This is also the case in lymphatic vessel invasion (ly-factor). Tumor cells in the ascites or pleural effusion are believed to represent late stage cancer (stage III or IV according to the WHO classification) [43].

The mechanisms involved in the intravasation of tumor cells have been intensively studied to date. Several histological investigations have been carried out to elucidate the mechanisms by which tumor cells enter blood vessels, lymphatic vessels, and coelomic cavities. These studies have identified the modalities of tumor cell intravasation; however, histological examinations using light microscopy have not yielded much information on the mechanisms of intravasation at the cellular level. In the 1970s, electron microscope began to be used in investigations of tumor metastasis, and together with the advances in immunohistology in the late 1980s, provided substantial information on the intravasation of tumor cells.

2.1. Migration into Blood Vessels

Microscopic investigations have revealed many differences in the features of intravasation of tumor cells by tumor types or by organs and tissues in which tumors arise. For straightforward examples, angiosarcoma and choriocarcinoma cells do not necessarily enter blood vessels to metastasize, because these malignant tumors are borne within blood vessels. Another example is the case where tumor cells enter an artery. Intravasation of tumor cells at the site of an artery is very rare, probably due to the presence of a dense fibromuscular covering.

However, it occurs frequently in lung cancer: Mosely et al. [44] reported arterial invasion in 11 of 25 cases (44%). We do not know why lung cancer cells, especially squamous cell carcinoma, frequently invade and enter pulmonary arteries. Many studies have demonstrated that almost all malignant tumors preferentially invade venous blood vessels, especially the small veins including the venules, and finally migrate into their lumen (Figure 15). Warren [45] demonstrated, using a transplantable melanoma in the cheek pouch membrane of golden hamster, that tumor cells are unlikely to invade the capillary sprouts migrating into the earliest tumor cell group during the initial angiogenesis phase or at the leading edge of the tumor because invasions into vessels of giant capillaries at the margin of tumors, capillaries with fenestrated endothelium, and capillaries with complete basement membranes are more likely.

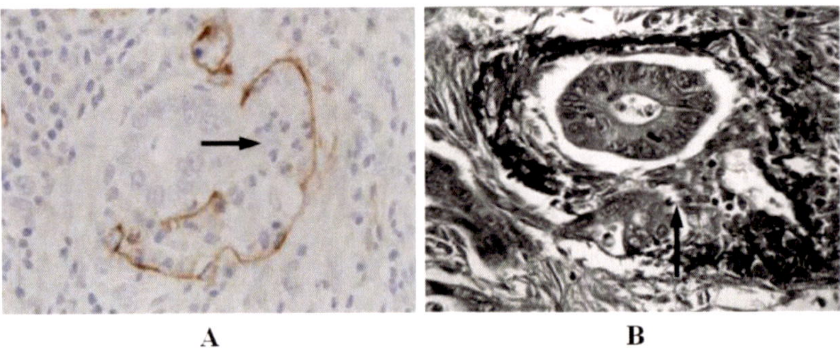

Figure 15. Intravasation of tumor cells. Intravasation of tumor cells in colorectal adenocarcinoma. A: Adenocarcinoma cells penetrating the vascular wall of a dilated giant capillary (arrow). Endothelial cells labeled with anti-CD31 antibody. B: Tumor cells invading and migrating into veins (arrow). Several cancer cells making gland (★) have entered the lumen (elastica-Masson stain).

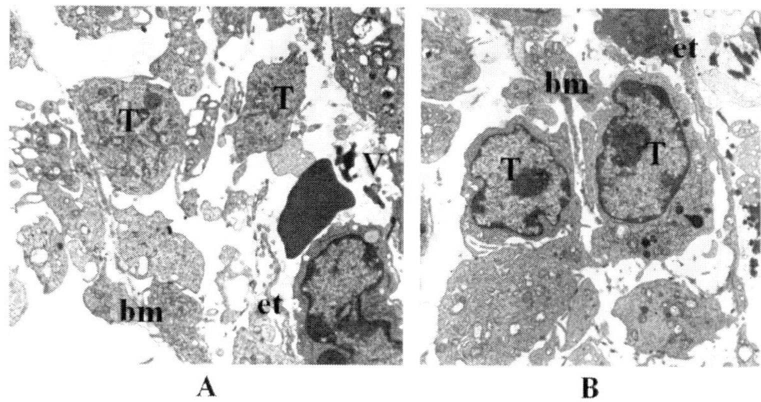

Figure 16. C3H mouse breast cancer cell (T) breaking through the basement membrane (bm) of an endothelial cell (et) and migrating into the capillary lumen [47].

In 1969, Kung et al. [46] presented the first transmission electron microscopic images of the migration of cancer cells into blood vessels. These images showed glioblastoma cells breaching the basement membrane of blood capillaries and migrating into the vascular lumen. Thereafter, several studies investigated the mechanism of tumor cell migration into blood vessels using different types of experimental tumor cells.

Some researchers, including ourselves, have demonstrated that tumor cells migrate into blood vessels via defect(s) created by themselves (Figure 16) [47]. On the other hands, Bruyn et al. [48] demonstrated that acute myelogenous leukemic cells penetrated the endothelial cell body by creating a temporary migration pore, which closed after the malignant cells had entered the vascular lumen.

Similar findings were reported by Azzarelli et al. [49], who studied the leptomeninges, a site of re-entry of leukemic cells into the systemic circulation. Constantinides et al. [50] found that fibrosarcoma cells caused the endothelial basement membrane to disappear and entered the venous lumen by inducing the opening of interendothelial junctions.

Another interesting type of intravasation is the development of tumor cells, which has been shown to be closely associated with the development of the vascular architecture (Figure 17) [51, 52]. Stromal cells in the perinecrotic area are immature and include active fibroblasts and myofibroblasts, and, in this case, the tumor vessels containing sprouts. The blood vessels are markedly dilated and appear to be sinusoidal and closely wrapped small tumor nests with vascular endothelial cells.

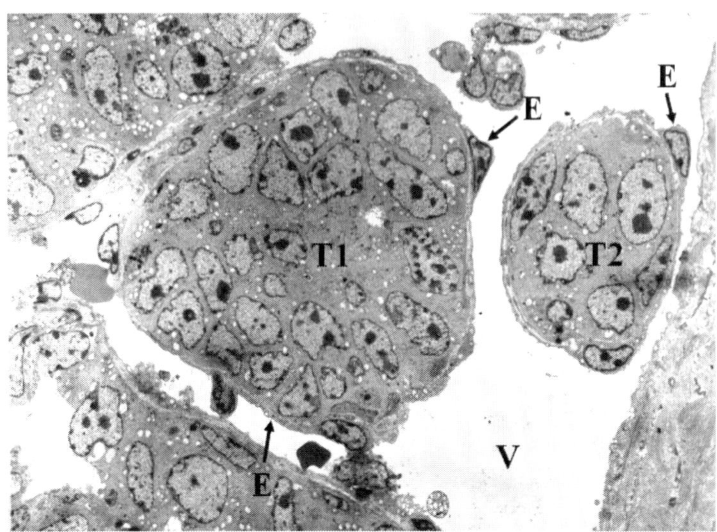

Figure 17. Intravasation of tumor cells in the primary site. Tumor nests (T1 and T2) of poorly differentiated carcinoma cells covered with vascular endothelial cells (E) appear floating in the sinusoidal vessels (V) [51].

Tumor cells then appear as tumor islands scattered in a sea of blood. These tumor nests encased in the vessel wall are then released into the circulation and transferred to the lung via the right cardiac system. Serial sections of the sinusoidal areas in several primary tumors have shown few floating nests of cells in the sinusoids that have no connection to the vascular walls. Therefore, we believe that there are two types of intravasation; active (or locomotive) and passive (or invasion-independent) [51, 53]. The active type of intravasation includes both destructive and non-destructive forms.

2.2. Migration into Lymphatic Vessels

In 1972, Takasawa [54] was the first to report the ultrastructures involved in intralymphatic migration of tumor cells. This study demonstrated destructive infiltration of lymphatic vessels due to implantation of an ascites hepatoma in the penile skin of rats. Araki [55] examined adenocarcinoma induced by *N*-methyl-*N'*-nitro-*N*-nitrosoguanidine in the stomach of a rat using electron microscopy and reported staging mechanism of the tumor cell invasion into the lymphatic vessel. In the first stage, tumor cells approached the lymphatic vessels and formed amoeba-like pseudopodia of tumor cells, which extended into amorphous perilymphatic space towards the lymphatic vessel. In the second stage, the microstructure of the cells moved into the lymphatic vessel, and in the final stage, the tumor cells proliferated in the lymphatic vessel and formed a cell cluster. Ultrastructural studies of human cancers were performed by Deutsch et al. [56], who reported that melanoma cells penetrate subendothelial space as single cells that then fuse with the endothelial cytoplasmic membrane and subsequently destroy the endothelial wall. In addition to this destructive migration, Carr et al. [57] reported a cytoplasmic process, wherein initially few cancer cells penetrated an open gap between endothelial cells followed by a mass of tumor cell cytoplasm. In addition, Paku et al. [58] found diapedesis-like intralymphatic migration of BSp73ASML cells (anaplastic sarcoma).

We were the first to describe passive intralymphatic migration of tumor cells [59]. Yoshida sarcoma (YS) cells are known to appear in circulating blood shortly after their intraperitoneal (ip) injection. We investigated the route and process of intravasation of YS cells using electron microscopy. Following 6 h–12 h after ip injection, YS cells were found in omental milky spots, which were enlarged by the presence of neutrophil leucocytes. At 24 h, in almost all cases, areas of the peritoneum lacking milky spots were not affected. YS cells proliferate solely in the milky spots to form tumor nodules with vascularization. However, intralymphatic involvement of YS cells is sometimes found within 24 h of inoculation. The endothelial cells show increased numbers of cytoplasmic organelle and cytoplasmic outgrowths, which usually contain few organelles and protrude into either the lumen or the interstitium. The cytoplasmic processes of the endothelial cells extend toward the surface of the YS cells and completely surround them. As a result, the YS cells appear to be enclosed within the endothelial cells (Figure 18).

The "milky spot" is an interesting site that contributes to the spread of tumor cells in the body [60]. This is because milky spots are associated with extramedullary hematopoiesis [61]. Milky spots fundamentally represent lymphoid tissue in the peritoneal cavity and are seen in the greater omentum, mesocolon, and the pouch of Douglas. They are composed of numerous macrophages and lymphocyte aggregates (omentum-associated lymphoid tissue). The lymphatic system of the greater omentum in animals, including humans, originates from the capillary lymphatics of the milky spots, where lymphatic endothelial cells form connections with milky spot mesothelial cells. Thus, capillary lymphatics in milky spots open within the abdominal cavity, and therefore tumor cells in the abdominal cavity can enter lymphatics in milky spots without any invasive migration. Except for our study described above, no studies on the intravasation/extravasation of tumor cells in milky spots have been performed to date, and there have been no reports on the mechanisms of intravasation of hematopoietic cells. Therefore, we are not convinced of the validity of our interpretation on the electron microscopic features, except that the mode of intravasation appears to resemble the transendothelial passage of tumor cells from the extravascular matrix in the lumen of absorbing lymphatic, as reported by Azzali [62]. Further studies should be conducted to validate this theory, because intravasation of cancer cells in the milky spots of the omentum is a crucial factor in the spread of cancer within the abdominal wall.

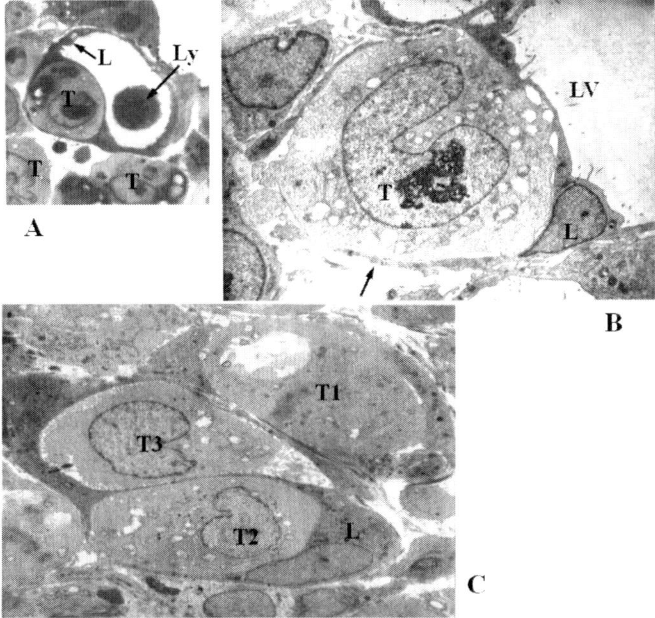

Figure 18. Intravasation of YS cells. A: YS cell (T) being enclosed by lymphatic endothelial cells (L) of a lymphatic vessel in a milky spot of the great omentum 24 h after intraperitoneal (ip) injection of tumor cells. Ly: Lymphocyte. Toluidine blue staining of a semi-ultrathin section of Epon-embedded material. B: Ultrastructural image of close contact between a YS cell and lymphatic endothelial cell (L). The YS cell appears to be enclosed by an elongated endothelial cell cytoplasmic protrusion. LV: Lymphatic vessel. C: Two YS cells (T2, T3) are surrounded by endothelial cells, and one YS cell (T1) is present in the lymphatic lumen [59]. Comment: We believed that the YS cells were in intravasation, but it might be also possible that the cells were in the process of extravasation.

2.3. Migration into Coelomic Cavity

Migration of tumor cells into the coelomic cavity appears to occur in a similar way to that of intralymphatic migration wherein cancer cells invade the basement membrane-like structure and mesothelial cell layer. However, there have been no detailed studies on the migration of cancer cells into the coelomic cavity except for that by Kobayashi et al. [63], who studied dissemination of tumor cells (rat ascites hepatoma AH130) into the peritoneum by invasion through the mesothelial lining. Their scanning electron microscopic study demonstrated that marked deformed tumor cells passed through a very small hole created in the peritoneum of peripheral areas of the tumor (Figure 19).

2.4. Mechanisms Involved in Tumor Intravasation

A. Mode of Intravasation; Active and Passive Intravasation

As described above, there are two types of intravasation from the morphological aspect; active and passive intravasation. In active intravasation, tumor cells migrate into the vascular lumina mainly by their own movement accompanied by some vascular wall destruction, which appears to be caused by active intrusion of cytoplasmic protrusions, such as pseudopodia and microvilli. This process is now well accepted and has been validated by several researchers, as described before.

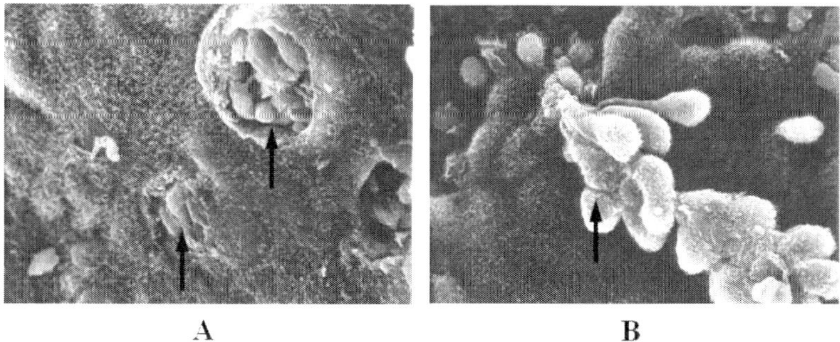

A B

Figure 19. Scanning electron micrographs of the migration of tumor cells into the peritoneal cavity. A: Tumor cells are seen in defects in the peritoneal wall (↑). B: Tumor cells in the abdominal wall entering the abdominal cavity (↑). These images were taken on the 11th day after inoculation of AH130 cells into the rectus abdominis muscle [63].

In contrast, some types of tumor cells, such as leukemia and malignant lymphoma, enter blood and lymphatic vessels through migration pores that have been created at intercellular junctions or through the extended cytoplasm of capillary endothelium. These pores appear to close after several tumor cells have passed through them. We call this active intravasation (Figure 20A).

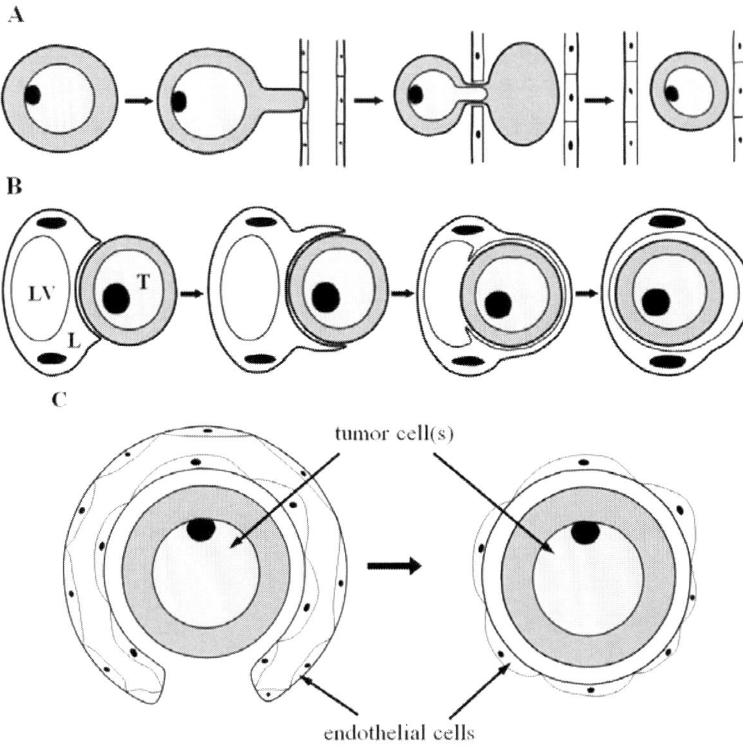

Figure 20. Schematic representation of tumor cell intravasation. A: Tumor cells adhere to endothelial cells of blood vessels/lymphatic vessels or mesothelial cells. Thereafter, these tumor cells migrate into vascular lumen or coelomic cavity through the defects of endothelial cells or mesothelial cells, which are made by tumor cells. Some types of tumor cells also are able to enter vascular lumen or coelomic cavity, through the opened intercellular junction or intracellular pathway of vascular endothelial cells or mesothelial cells. B: Transport of tumor cell into vascular cavity. Endothelial cells (L) extend cytoplasmic protrusions to tumor cell(s) and then enclose them entirely. The cytoplasmic process of endothelial cells at locations facing the lumen (LV) disappears, which results in translocation of tumor cells in the lumen. C: A tumor cell or tumor cell cluster is enclosed by vascular endothelial cells. The tissue fragment, which is composed of vascular tissues and tumor cell(s), is released into vascular lumen and transported. Similar phenomenon will occur in coelomic wall.

Intravasation by tumor cells can also occur through active movement of the endothelial cells of blood and lymphatic vessels, by which tumor cells appear to be transported into the vascular lumen. We have termed the process passive intravasation. Furthermore, tumor cells appear to be involved in the remodeling of blood vessels, also resulting in passive intravasation. Pathologists have observed the release of tumor cells growing in blood vessels in renal cell carcinoma, hepatocellular carcinoma, and thyroid cancers. These modes of intravasation may be corresponding to passive type of intravasation [64]. Interestingly, Nakanishi et al. [65] hypothesized the basement membrane fusion of tumor cells and vascular endothelial cells in tumor cell intravasation. These latter types of intravasation will be seen in Figure 20 classified as passive type of intravasation (Figure 20B, C).

B. Molecules in Tumor Cell Intravasation

Similar to some workers [66-68], we consider that mechanism(s) involved in the adhesion of tumor cells and vascular components including endothelial cells and the basement membrane component(s) is of absolute importance for tumor cell intravasation, although other components, such as chemotactic /haptotactic factors, and degradation enzymes for extravascular matrices are also important. For example, tumor cell intravasation occurs not only in connective tissues surrounding tumor but also within cancer tissues, suggesting that locomotion/hepatotaxis is not crucial for tumor cell intravasation. Therefore, we investigated the adhesion molecules including carbohydrates of tumor cells over a long period of time in relation to intravasation [53, 69-74] (Section III, in detail), as seen in the following two studies, the first of which was of human breast cancer. Since metastasis is intimately associated with the interaction of tumor cells and host tissues, especially with respect to cell surface adhesion molecules including carbohydrates, we examined the relationship between the carbohydrate expression of tumor cells in primary and lymph node metastasis in breast cancer. In another recent study, we investigated aberrant MUC1 bearing the Tn antigen of rat ascites hepatoma AH109A cells (poorly differentiated hepatocellular carcinoma) with a strong lymphatic metastatic propensity [72]. These cells metastasized to lymph nodes two to three weeks following inoculation into the subcutaneous tissues of the abdominal wall when intercellular adhesion molecule-1 (ICAM-1) appeared in the vascular walls around the tumor.

At present, we do not know how human breast tumor cells migrate into lymphatic vessels and how the (approximately) 33 kDa aberrant MUC1 bearing the Tn antigen plays a role on intravasation into lymphatic vessels. However, it can be stated that tumor cells that strongly express MUC1 frequently embolize in the lymphatic vessels. MUC1 bearing the Tn antigen may interact with ICAM-1 on endothelial cells, as suggested by Rhan et al. [75]. Furthermore, recently, Danussi et al. [76] reported that a newly generated functional antibody had identified Tn antigen as a novel determinant in the tumor cell-lymphatic endothelium interaction. More detailed description will appear in Chapter III, Section 3.

We do not know the molecular mechanisms of passive type tumor cell intravasation that was observed in milky spot of the ometum. The mechanism of transendothelial passage of tumor cells, which was claimed by Azzali, also remains to be unclear [77]. On the other hand, recently, Sugino et al. [78] identified the secretory leukocyte protease inhibitor (SLPI) as a candidate gene responsible for passive type intravasation (Figure 20, C; the authors called it an invasion-independent pathway). They then studied the functional role of SPLI in metastatic dissemination by transfecting the SLPI gene into a poorly metastatic clone of the MCH66 mouse mammary tumor cell line. Over-expression of SLPI promoted in vivo growth and spontaneous metastasis to the lung, whereas it suppressed invasive activity in vitro. The inoculated tumors of SLPI-transfectants exclusively induced a sinusoidal vasculature and subsequently produced endothelially coated emboli, which are morphological indices of the invasion-independent pathway. Furthermore, exogenous SLPI inhibited the migration activity through the migration activity through matrigel of tumor and human umbilical vein endothelial cells. In vivo angiogenesis assays also demonstrated that SLPI suppressed the migration of newly formed blood vessels. These authors also claimed that an anti-migratory effect of SLPI on tumor-associated endothelial cells may induce vascular remodeling to form a sinusoidal architecture and consequently promote invasion-independent metastasis.

Fundamentally, tumor cells proliferate expansively and move at random and encounter blood and lymphatic vessels, but these movements do not explain the preferential intravasation of these cells into small veins including post-capillary venules and/or lymphatic vessels. Specific factor(s) may be involved in this process. Thrombus may be a specific mediator because this is frequently seen in veins in primary cancer. Platelets promote locomotion of some types of tumor cells as seen in microcinetography analysis (see next section). Another interesting factor concerns the amount of chemotactic factor associated with smooth muscle cells that constitute veins. Navigation by neurotransmitters may be involved in intravasation of tumor cells [79].

Chemokine receptors of cancer cells, such that of CXCR4 and CCCR7, are interested in some kinds of cancer cell intravasation. Chemokines are a superfamily of small, cytokine-like proteins that induce, through their interaction with G-protein-coupled receptor, cytoskeletal rearrangement, firm adhesion to endothelial cells and directional migration [80]. It is likely that organ-preference metastasis of some kinds of cancer such breast cancer and malignant melanoma can be explained at least in part by the presence of chemokine receptors of these tumor cells.

3. Transport: Significance and Fate of Circulating Tumor Cells

Transport of tumor cells is a critical event that discriminates between invasion and metastasis. In general, it is said that this process causes significant tumor cell death, with 99.9% or more cells dying within 24 h of entry in circulation [81, 82]. Quite simply, metastatic tumor cells have a capacity to escape cell death during transport. Our current understanding of tumor cell death during transport is that it varies among tumor types and routes of transport, namely hematogenous, lymphatic, and/or coelomic transport [83, 84]. At this point, we would like to stress that the fate of tumor cells in the circulation, in addition to tumor cell death, is related to two crucial properties of the metastatic phenomenon: organ affinity and metastatic potential.

3.1. Factors Affecting Tumor Cell Survival or Death During Transport

Luscher [85] described how certain types of tumor cells were killed when they were introduced into the bloodstream. To date, several types of serum protein (antibody, complement, blood coagulation activity, and lipoprotein) and cells (natural killer cells, cytotoxic killer cells, and neutrophils) have been demonstrated as having the capacity to kill tumor cells in specific ways [86, 87].

Deformation is considered to be an important component of cellular character relating to cancer cell circulation in the blood [88, 89]. Sato et al. [88] demonstrated that poor deformed tumor cells were not viable after one passage through the pulmonary blood vessels. We [90] examined the influence of fluid flow on tumor cells using a newly devised circulation system (Figure 21) and demonstrated that Yoshida sarcoma cells and two rat ascites tumor cell lines (AH130 and AH7974) remained viable up to 72-96 h in a 10 mm-diameter tube in the circulation apparatus at a speed of 1.0 meter (m)/second (s) and that these cells retained their experimental metastatic potential to a similar or greater degree when compared with those cells cultured outside the circulation (Table 1). These results suggest that circulating rat ascites hepatoma cells in the blood suffer little mechanical damage from fluid flow.

Transport of tumor cells to distant tissues/organs implies that these cells lose their supporting substrates. This loss of substrate may affect the fate of tumor cells in the body in at least two different ways, the first being cell death in the circulation. In general, cell-matrix interactions have major effects on phenotypic features such as gene regulation, differentiation, and cell growth control.

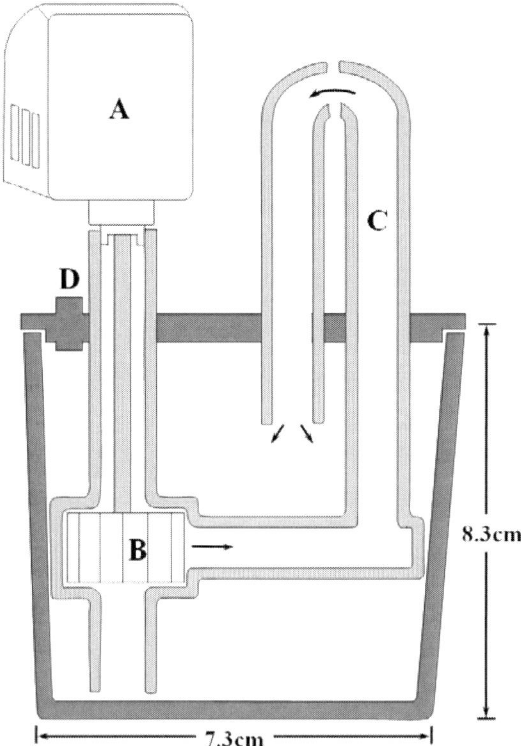

Figure 21. Circulating apparatus. A: motor, B: propeller, C: circulatory tube, D: pore for injection or aspiration of cell suspension [90].

Table 1. Comparison of experimental metastatic potential of non-circulating and circulating tumor cells

Time after circulation (h)	Fluid flow (m/s)	No. of animals died with tumors/total no. of animals examined (%)		
		Yoshida sarcoma	AH 130	AH 7974
0	0	13/18 (72%)	5/15 (33%)	6/8 (75%)
6	0	14/18 (77%)	5/12 (42%)	5/8 (63%)
	1.0	12/20 (60%)	3/15 (20%)	6/8 (75%)
24	0	7/8 (88%)	3/14 (21%)	6/9 (67%)
	1.0	6/9 (66%)	9/14 (64%)	7/10 (70%)

One milliliter of tumor cell suspension (2-15 × 10^4 cells/ml) circulated at a speed of 1.0 m/s or cultured in a test tube (0 m/s) for a fixed period was injected into the tail vein of rats. All animals were autopsied at the time of death or 100 days after the injection [90].

Disruption of the epithelial cell-matrix interaction induces apoptosis (anoikis), and many studies have demonstrated that circulating tumor cells are frequently apoptotic [91]. Some recent studies suggest that (1) Src (a non-receptor protein kinase) plays an essential role in the development of apoptosis resistance in various tumors [92], and (2) metastatic tumor cells in circulating blood possess a particular Src signal transduction system that facilitates avoidance of cell death.

Another theory is the drastic enhancement of the metastatic potential of certain types of tumor cells through anchor loss, as reported by Raz et al. [93], who studied lung colonization of B16-F1 cells grown in a flat or spherical configuration. These authors discovered that the cells cultivated in vitro as spheroids on a non-adhesive substrate reversibly expressed a marked increase in their propensity to establish metastasis and that the altered metastatic capability was accompanied by both a reversible reduction in the accessibility of cell surface proteins to external iodination and a dramatic increase in the synthesis of vimentin.

Cell shape may play a critical role in growth control. It was postulated that signals from the environment could regulate various cellular activities that may affect the metastatic properties of the cells. As reported by Folkman et al. [94], cell shape was found to be tightly coupled to DNA synthesis and growth in non-transformed cells. Gonda et al. [95] recently demonstrated that protease-activated receptor 1 (PAR1) movement on cell membranes increases during intravasation, reaches a peak within the vessel, and decreases during extravasation.

Thus, acquisition of anchor-independent growth seems to be a prerequisite feature of metastatic cells, but establishment of its molecular nature requires further studies.

3.2. Evidence of Circulating Tumor Cells in the Body

In the early 1950s, circulation of tumor cells throughout the body following intravasation was a major point of debate with respect to tumor metastasis. The reason for this uncertainty was the fact that, in general, tumor cells are too large to pass through capillary beds since the majority of tumor cells are larger than both erythrocytes and leukocytes. It was therefore reasoned that secondary metastasis must occur via the passage of tumor cells through arterio-venous shunts or an atrial septal defect. In 1952, Zeidman and Buss [96] first demonstrated that tumor cells are able to pass through pulmonary blood vessels, and Moore et al. [97] reported circulated tumor cells in peripheral blood. Nakamura et al. [98] demonstrated that rat ascites hepatoma AH13 cells pass more rapidly through the blood vessels of the lower extremity than any of the organs examined, followed by the kidney and then the liver.

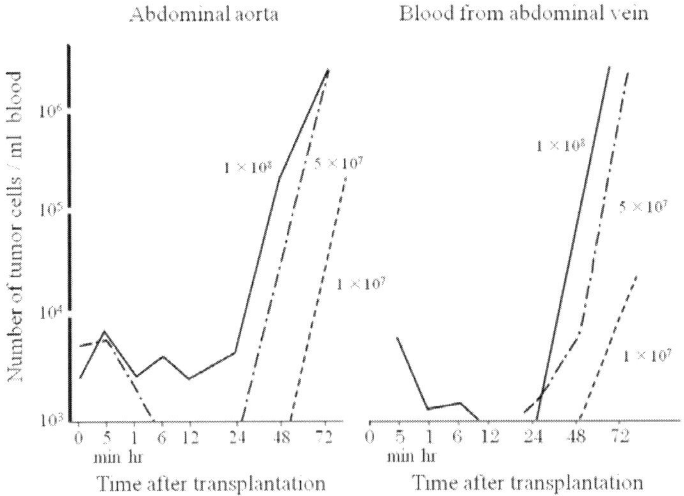

Figure 22. Circulating tumor cells in the blood. Yoshida sarcoma cells were injected into rat tail veins. The cells subsequently were collected by the Conrey-Ficoll method and were counted. Tumor cells had disappeared by 6 -24 h after injection, and thereafter a striking number of tumor cells appeared in the blood [99].

The lungs offered maximum resistance to the passage of tumor cells. We followed their observation (Figure 22). Recent studies using polymerase chain reaction and positron emission topography have clearly demonstrated that tumor cells in the blood of advanced-stage patients circulate throughout whole body, albeit to different degrees depending on tumor type. This is also true in the case of tumor cells within the lymphatic vessels and coelomic cavity.

We believe that circulating tumor cells have two roles in metastasis; one is that more tumor cells in the circulation will encounter more tissues suitably fertile soil for their metastasis, and the other is that circulating tumor cells are able to injure microcirculation systems and tissues. These microinjuries followed by tissue repair may provide fertile soil for their metastasis. We will discuss this in Chapter II in detail.

4. Lodgement: First Step of Tumor Cell Implantation

In the case of tumor metastasis, it is generally accepted that successful implantation consists of three sequential steps; lodgment, extravasation, and early growth, although sometimes no distinct border exists between them in terms of cellular behavior and growth kinetics.

4.1. Kinetics of Lodgment and Proliferation

Lodgment of circulating tumor cells was discovered by Wood in 1958 [100], who observed V2 carcinoma cells in the circulation of the ear chamber by microcinematography. Sato and Suzuki [101] followed his investigations by observing the fate of rat ascites tumor cells (AH66F, AH601) in rat mesenteric microcirculation. These authors stressed the importance of adhesion of cancer cells to endothelial cells in the lodgment of tumor cells in the microcirculation.

Although lodgment of tumor cell emboli is undoubtedly a fundamental prerequisite to metastasis formation, the outcome and incidence of metastases are not determined by this factor alone. Therefore, we carried out experimental studies to define the kinetics of cell arrest and proliferation, using rat ascites hepatoma cell line AH7974 and its variant subline AH7974F [102-104]. These two cell lines are useful experimental tools for studying not only the incidence of brain metastasis but also the factors that may influence the anatomic location of metastatic growth. They produce completely different patterns of metastatic distribution within the brain, independent of the route of cell injection. When inoculated via the carotid artery, AH7974 cells produce experimental metastases in the brain parenchyma, meninges, and choroid plexus but do not establish colonies in the liver. In contrast, AH7974F cells produce infiltrative growth in the liver but minimal tumor growth in the brain parenchyma. As shown in Figures 23 and 24, the number of tumor cells arrested in the brain and liver varies significantly between the two cell lines. AH7974 cells, which are highly effective in colonizing the brain, are arrested in the blood vessels of the brain, undergo rapid disappearance (6 h), and very few cells remain lodged in the blood vessels after 12–48 h. Although proliferation of tumor cells was evident 12 h after injection, the period of maximum cell proliferation in the brain parenchyma did not occur until 72 h after initial arrest. Strikingly, tumor cells were not detected in the liver at any time. In contrast, AH7974F cells, which colonize the liver but not the brain, showed a similar rapid decrease in the number of embolic tumor cells in the brain in the first 6 h after injection, followed by slow disappearance over 72 h. However, no evidence of extravasation or cell proliferation could be detected. In the liver, however, the AH7974F cells proliferated rapidly and infiltrated into the parenchyma.

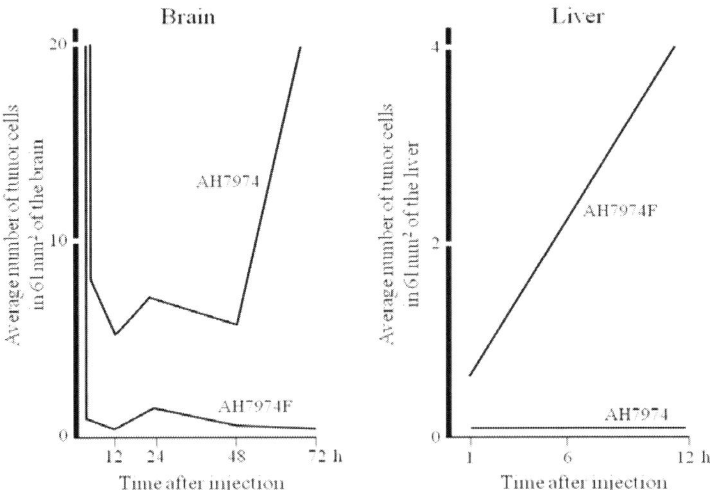

Figure 23. Arrest and proliferation of rat ascites hepatoma AH7974 and AH7974F cells in rat brain and liver after injection via the internal carotid artery [102].

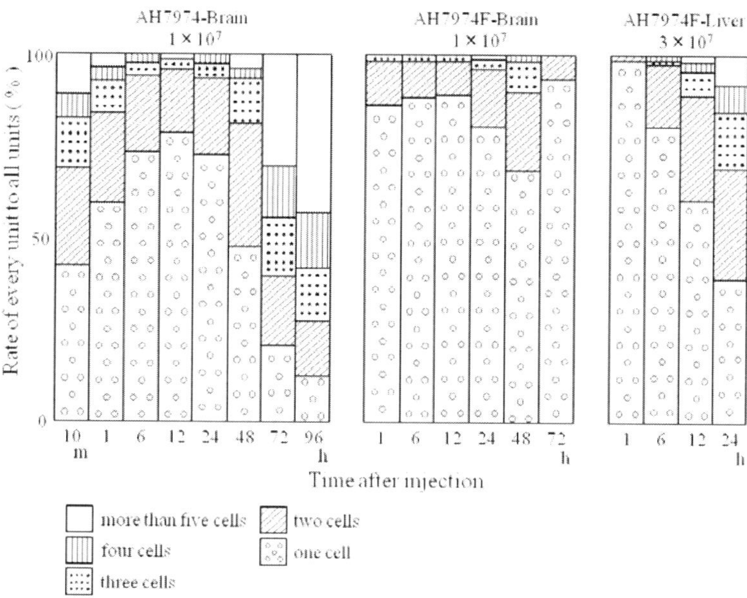

Figure 24. Proliferation kinetics of rat ascites hepatoma AH7974 and AH7974F cells arrested in the brain and liver after injection via the internal carotid artery. The number of tumor cells contained in a unit of tissue (0.61 mm^2 in sections ~3 μm thick) was examined [104].

Using tritiated thymidine ([^{3}H] TdR) autoradiography, the flash-labeling index of AH7974 cells in the brain ranged from 10% to 30% six h after tumor injection. Over the next one to five days, the labeling indices ranged from 41% to 55% and then declined to approximately 20% by seven days. In animals receiving multiple injections of [^{3}H]TdR, the labeling indices for tumor cells in the brain parenchyma increased progressively after injection and reached about 90% after 24 h. The labeling indices of tumor cells in the choroid plexus were even higher: in flash-labeling experiments, labeling indices ranging from 54% to 79% were observed and in continuous-labeling experiments, the labeling index reached 96% 24 h after tumor injection (Table 2). In contrast, flash labeling of AH7974F cells in the brain yielded maximum values ranging from 31% to 55% at 48 h after tumor injection, but even after multiple [^{3}H]TdR doses, the labeling index did not increase. In the same animals, flash-labeling indices for tumor cells in the liver ranged from 61% to 75% 48 h post injection, and continuous labeling indices had reached 92% by 12 h post injection (Table 3). These data are also supported by observations made with isotope dilution methods and direct counts of radioactive silver granule labeling indices. The average number of silver granules per tumor cell detected in the brain did not decrease with time after the injection of tumor cells, but the average number of silver granules in tumor cells trapped initially in the liver declined to half and to one quarter at 24 and 48 h, respectively (Figure 25).

Table 2. Labeling index of AH7974 cells with [^{3}H]TdR after arrest in different regions of the central nervous system

	Time after injection	Labeling index of tumor cells			
		Brain parenchyman		Choroid plexux	
		Mean	SD (n)	Mean	SD (n)
Flash labeling	6 h *	23.8	11.2(3)	57.9	3.0(3)
	1 day *	43.6	2.6(3)	61.8	5.3(3)
	2 days *	50.5	1.8(2)	63.0	5.3(2)
	3 days *	51.2	4.0(3)	74.6	8.4(3)
	4 days *	50.0	4.3(2)	67.2	0.7(2)
	5 days *	46.5	1.5(2)	64.3	9.5(2)
	7 days	22.5	0.8(2)	-	-
Continuous labeling	6 h *	68.4	0.6(2)	85.4	3.7(2)
	12 h *	74.0	9.8(3)	94.1	1.5(3)
	1 day *	86.6	0.4(2)	96.9	1.5(3)
	2 days *	89.5	3.5(2)	99.0	1.0(2)
	3 days	96.6	3.7(2)	100.0	0.0(3)

* There was a statistical significance in the labeling indices between tumor cells in the brain and in the choroid plexus ($p < 0.01$).

Table 3. Labeling index of AH7974F cells with [^{3}H]TdR arrested in brain and liver

	Time after injection(h)	Labeling index of tumor cells			
		Brain		Liver	
		Mean	SD (n)	Mean	SD (n)
Flash labeling	1 *	47.5	3.9(2)	64.5	3.2(2)
	6	58.0	1.8(3)	61.0	1.4(3)
	12 *	30.5	17.5(2)	69.5	1.8(2)
	24 *	44.5	0.3(3)	68.7	2.9(3)
	48 *	52.0	2.1(2)	75.0	1.4(3)
Continuous labeling	6 *	60.6	2.4(3)	75.3	2.1(3)
	12 *	48.0	0.4(3)	91.6	1.4(3)
	24 *	47.3	6.0(2)	89.5	1.8(2)

* There was a statistical significance in the labeling indexes between tumor cells in the brain and liver ($p < 0.01$).

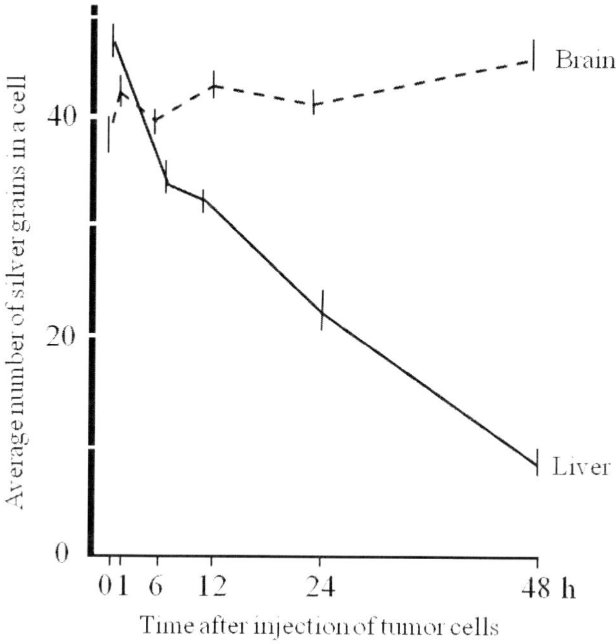

Figure 25. Average number of silver granules in tumor cells labeled with [^{3}H] TdR [103].

These results indicate that AH7974 cells injected via the carotid artery were able to arrest in the cerebral capillaries, initiate proliferation, and then extravasate into the brain parenchyma and renew proliferation to establish metastatic foci. On the other hand, AH7974F cells that arrested in brain vessels remained viable but ceased dividing, while cells from the same inocula that embolized liver sinusoids initiated rapid proliferation. We therefore conclude that the fate of embolic tumor cells was influenced strongly by the microenvironment in which they were arrested. When circulating cells are arrested in a suitable organ, they can migrate into perivascular tissue and proliferate, but when lodged in hostile sites, they are either unable to extravasate, or if they do extravasate, they are unable to proliferate to establish a metastatic lesion.

4.2. Mechanisms Involved in Arrest and Lodgement

The factors associated with lodgment of tumor cells in the microcirculation have been studied extensively, but consensus as to the mechanisms involved has still to be reached. Mechanical, thrombotic, and electrostatic phenomena have been proposed as important elements of host (patho)physiology affecting this process, together with the possible role of specific tumor cell components in determining tumor cell arrest patterns [105, 106]. However, once again, the respective importance of each of these factors in any given tumor or tissue site is unknown.

To examine the morphological features of tumor cell lodgment in blood vessels, we undertook extensive ultrastructural observations to compare tumor models in which metastasis appears to be explained primarily by the anatomical–mechanical hypothesis to those in which the seed and soil hypothesis appears to be more influential [35-37, 107,108] (see Chapter II). We consider that lodgment of tumor cells in the microcirculation occurs via three nonexclusive mechanisms: 1) direct attachment of tumor cells to vascular endothelial cells; 2) direct adhesion of tumor cells to the subendothelial basement membrane; and 3) entrapment of tumor cells within thrombi found in the vessel lumen.

The adhesion of circulating tumor cells to vascular endothelial cells as an active process has been proposed by Warren et al. [109, 110], Cotmore and Carter [111], and Sindelar et al. [112]. In our observations on rat ascites hepatoma cell lines, the initial interactions occur by the formation of cell-to-cell contacts in which the plasma membranes of the interacting cells are separated by a gap of about 100 Å. This type of junctional contact was frequently seen at the tips of cytoplasmic processes extending from the surfaces of the opposing cells (Figures 26, 27). The cytoplasm beneath the plasma membrane in certain such contact regions contained fine fibrous materials about 50 Å in diameter. Formation of tight contacts of this kind did not increase the electron opacity of the intercellular space and the subjacent cytoplasm in either tumor cells or endothelial cells. The contacts formed in these situations resemble those described in numerous previous studies of cell adhesion [113, 114]. The formation of organized junctional structures, such as tight or gap junctions or desmosomes, was not observed. A second type of contact observed with regular frequency involves the interdigitation and insertion of tumor cell protrusions into the coated and non-coated vesicles of adjacent cells. Similar findings have been observed by Roos et al. [115, 116] and Dingemans et al. [117] in tumor cell colonization of the liver.

Adhesion of tumor cells to regions of exposed subendothelial basement membrane in blood vessels is seen at sites of tumor cell arrest with both high- and low-organ preference metastatic profiles (Figure 28). For example, cells of the brain-colonizing AH7974 cell line attached to exposed regions of basement membrane were frequently seen in cerebral capillaries three days after injection of tumor cells [108].

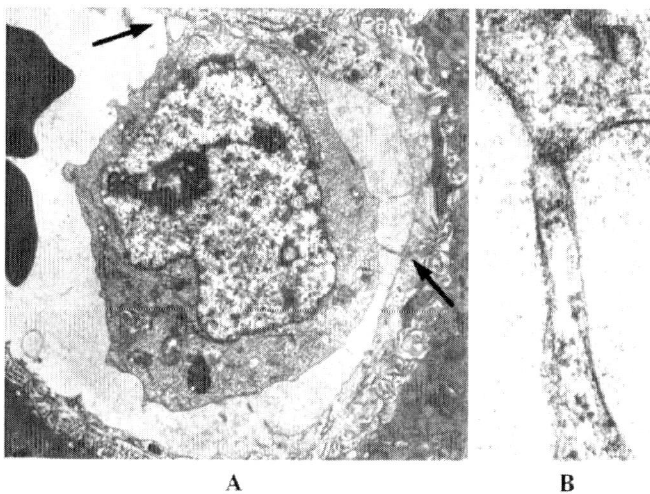

Figure 26. A: A Yoshida sarcoma cell in liver sinusoid in contact with an endothelial cell at the tips of its cytoplasmic processes (↑). B: Higher magnification of the contact region [21].

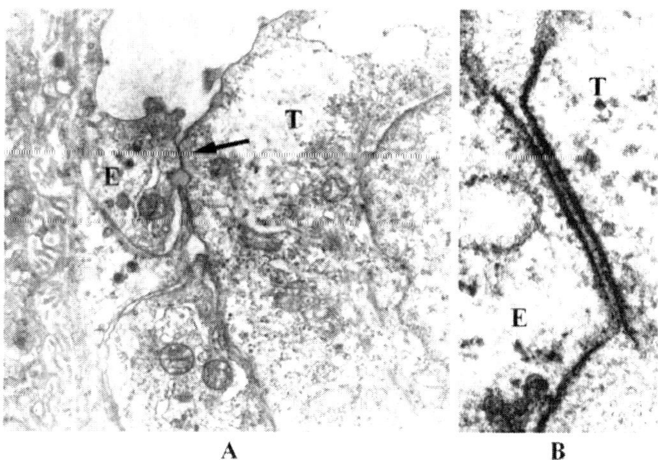

Figure 27. A: AH7974F cell in liver sinusoid, attached to endothelial cell (arrowhead). B: Higher magnification of the contact region; the opposing cell membranes show a parallel and straight arrangement across a gap of about 100 Å. E: endothelial cell, T: tumor cell [21].

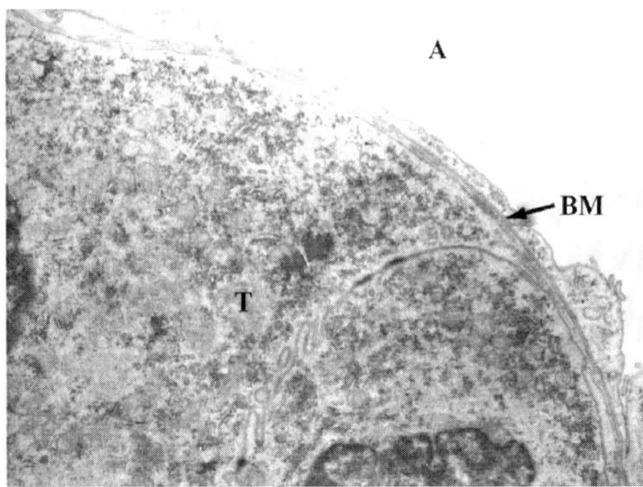

Figure 28. Arrested rat ascites hepatoma 601 cells adhered to basal lamina of pulmonary capillary. A: alveolar lumen, BM: basement membrane, T: tumor cells [107].

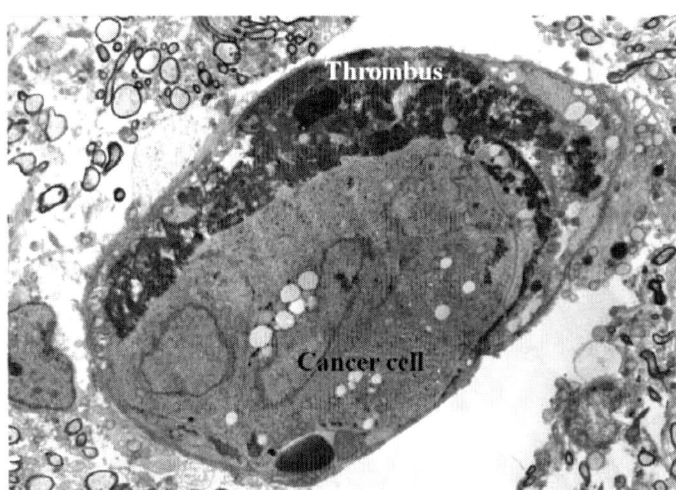

Figure 29. Rat ascites hepatoma AH7974 cells embedded in brain blood vessel [Kawaguchi T, unpublished data].

Similarly, Wallace et al. [118] and Kinjyo [119] reported that Walker 256 cells and AH130 cells, respectively, adhered to the basement membrane of pulmonary capillaries 6 h after the injection of tumor cells.

Many workers have reported an association between thrombus formation and tumor cell lodgment in the microvasculature (Figure 29) [118-120]. The importance of platelet aggregation and thrombus formation as a site for tumor cell arrest varies substantially between tumors and at different body sites. For example, the lodgment of Yoshida sarcoma cells and AH7974F and AH13 hepatoma cells in the liver sinusoids is rarely associated with thrombus formation [21]. This can probably be explained by the fact that the thromboplastic activities of these tumor cells and liver tissue are low. Similar findings on the lodgment of tumor cells in the liver were reported by Cotmore and Carter [111], Dingemans et al. [117], and Chew et al. [120].

We doubt whether thrombus formation precedes tumor cell lodgment, because fibrin thrombi and platelet aggregations are usually found surrounding tumor cells but not between tumor cells and the vascular wall. Secondly, fibrin and or/platelets usually disappear from the regions of tumor cells that are still lodged in the blood vessels. We do not consider that thrombus formation is necessary for tumor cells to lodge in blood vessels, though this may well have an important role in sequestering tumor cells from assault by host defenses, and in facilitating the retention of tumor cells that are weakly attached to the vascular wall within the microvasculature, in order that sufficient time be allowed for their extravasation.

5. Extravasation of Tumor Cells

5.1. Kinetics

Experimental studies suggest that the kinetics of extravasation for tumor cells varies among different organs and also differs significantly in different tumors. Detailed description is done in Ref. 37. Briefly, in the sinusoidal capillaries of the liver, tumor cells can migrate rapidly through the sinusoidal wall into the space of Disse and gain access to the hepatic cords within 24 h of injection [21, 115-117].

In contrast, tumor cell extravasation is significantly slower in organs lined by continuous capillaries because they present a more complex mechanical barrier to extravasation as a result of the endothelial architecture and presence of a basement membrane. Thus, tumor cell extravasation takes 24~48 h in the lung [112, 119, 120], and 48~72 h in the brain and in the renal glomeruli [107, 108, 120]. In addition, the intrinsic properties of the tumor cells themselves will also influence extravasation kinetics. We observed that AH130 cells were able to proliferate within glomerular capillaries to form colonies of sufficient size, but they undergo avascular necrosis without accomplishing extravasation, while AH7974 cells lodged in the same location migrated rapidly into Bowman's space [107].

5.2. Mechanisms of Tumor Cell Extravasation

The first detailed study of this topic was undertaken by Wood [100], who followed the fate of blood-borne V2 tumor cells in the ear chamber of a rabbit using continuous microcinematography. He found that defects in the structural integrity of the endothelial lining occurred when one or more leukocytes had passed through the vessel wall and that tumor cells were able to follow and emigrate into the surrounding connective tissue. Subsequently, many ultrastructural studies have been performed on the extravasation of tumor cells of diverse histologic lineages in a variety of animal organs. Despite this extensive body of work, the original report of Wood has still to be confirmed. In the meantime, two or three alternative mechanisms of tumor cell extravasation have been proposed [119- 123]. These include the diapedesis of single tumor cells, the migration of tumor cell emboli into the extravascular parenchyma at areas of damage to the vessel wall, and the invasion and breaching of the continuity of the endothelial cell lining by pseudopodal extensions generated by arrested tumor cells. Review of the available literature suggests that mechanisms used by different tumor cells in different experimental systems can vary, even within the same tissue.

We have studied the mode of extravasation of rat ascites hepatoma cells (AH13, AH7974F, AH601, AH7974) and Yoshida sarcoma cells in the brain, lung, liver, kidney, and adrenal glands. These observations have revealed three major patterns of extravasation [21, 35, 37, 107, 108].

A. Locomotion-Type Extravasation

In this form of extravasation, tumor cells lodged in capillaries or small veins migrate into the perivascular tissue through their own movement. Three general categories of migratory behavior have been identified.

First, tumor cells can migrate through the intercellular junctions between adjacent endothelial cells in a fashion analogous to the diapedesis of neutrophil leukocytes [124-126]. We have only occasionally observed gaps in the intercellular junctions between endothelial cells at sites of tumor cell arrest.

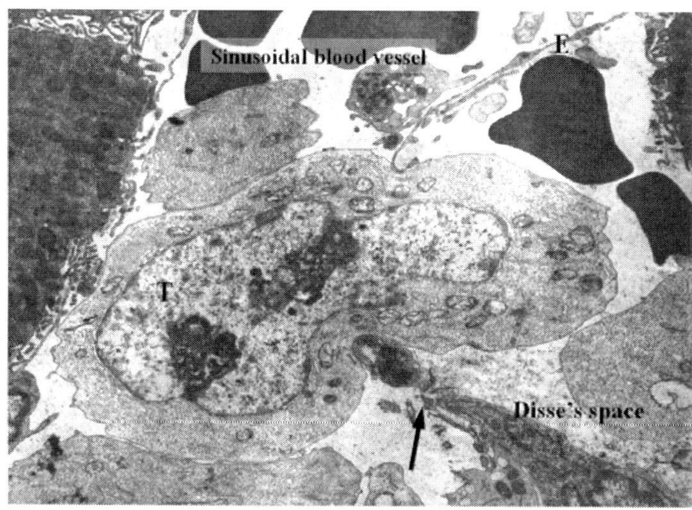

Figure 30. Extravasation of Yoshida sarcoma cell in liver sinusoid. T: Yoshida sarcoma cell. E: endothelial lining. Arrow shows the supposed endothelial cell junction [21].

A second pattern of locomotory extravasation involves transendothelial migration. The continuity of the endothelial cell surface in renal glomerular capillaries and liver sinusoids is interrupted by multiple pores and fenestrations and by a high degree of pinocytotic and endocytic activity. Rat ascites hepatoma cells can insert cytoplasmic processes into these openings and are apparently able to migrate through the endothelial cell to reach the extravascular compartment tissue, with no apparent damage to or destruction of endothelial cells (Figure 30). Extravasation of blood-borne lymphosarcoma cells and monocytes in liver sinusoids may occur by a similar mechanism.

The third mechanism involves migration of tumor cells through endothelial defects. This has been reported in numerous tissues following the arrest of tumor cells belonging to diverse histologic origins. The process appears to advance by the creation of endothelial defects as a consequence of direct attack by tumor cells. The nature and extent of the endothelial defects differ widely in different tumors and host tissues and also between tumor cells of the same type lodged in the vasculature of different organs. Endothelial cell degeneration and necrosis can also give rise to endothelial defects that serve as conduits for tumor cell extravasation. One of the more obvious events leading to endothelial cell degeneration and necrosis is the compression of the vessel by the proliferating tumor mass. We have reported this to be a common finding in liver sinusoids, but it is rare in cerebral capillaries. Retraction of endothelial cells caused by tumor cells appears to occur primarily at sites in which the endothelial cells are only weakly adherent to the underlying basement membrane and at sites that lack a distinct basement membrane. Tumor cells that lodge in segments of the microvasculature lacking an underlying basement membrane, such as the liver sinusoid, are able to achieve extravasation simply by penetrating through the endothelium. In contrast, tumor cells that can penetrate the basement membrane are a requirement of extravasation in vascular beds that possess basement membranes.

Analysis of extravasation of tumor cells arrested in cerebral capillaries has revealed that the first step in extravasation involves the appearance of small pores in the basement membrane in the immediate vicinity of tumor cells. This is followed by insertion of small tumor cell pseudopodia into these defects. Subsequently, the tips of the protruding pseudopodal processes become longer and swell into a balloon-like protrusion.

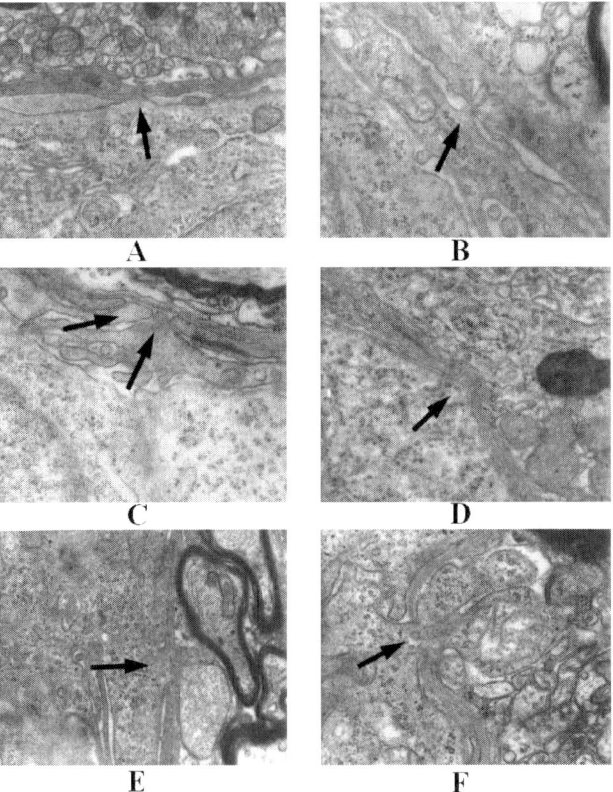

Figure 31. (continued).

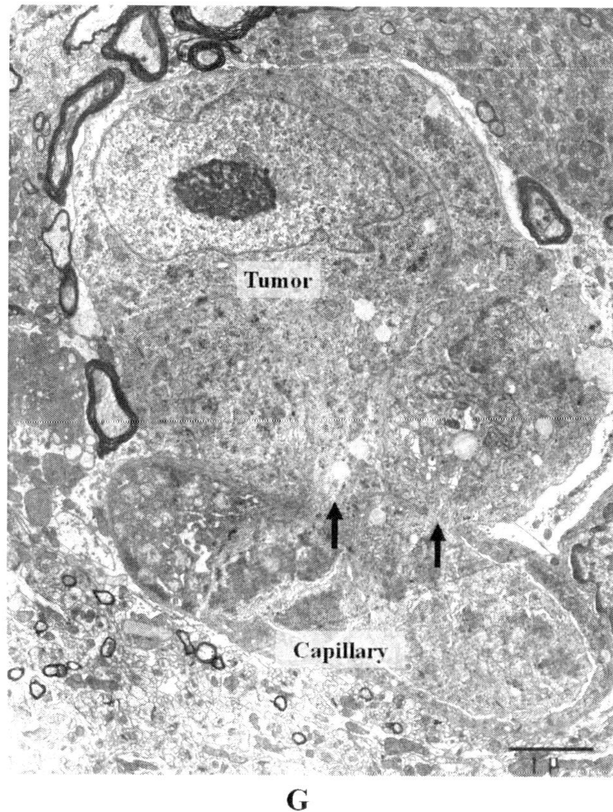

Figure 31. The assumed process of extravasation of rat ascites hepatoma AH7974 cells in the rat brain. A: An AH7974 cell process (arrowhead) has penetrated the vascular endothelium three days post-injection. B: The tip of the tumor cell process (arrowhead) has inserted into the vascular endothelium three days post-injection. The endothelium appears to have detached slightly from the underlying basal lamina. C: Two tumor cell pseudopodia (arrowheads) have pushed aside the endothelial cells three days post-injection. The intercellular junction between the endothelial cells and basal lamina appears to be almost intact. D: A tumor cell adheres to the basement membrane of the blood vessel (arrowhead). E: A tumor cell projects its balloon-like pseudopodium into the perivascular tissue through a small pore (diameter, 0.61 μm) in the basal lamina at an early stage (three days) of extravasation. The basement membrane is destroyed, through which an AH7974 cell pseudopodium is protruding into the extravascular portion (arrowhead). F: At three days post-injection, extravascular protrusions from a tumor cell containing glycogen granules and rough endoplasmic reticulum membranes is seen (arrowhead), but no mitochondria are noted. G: Extravasating AH7974 cells have migrated through two pores (arrows) in the capillary wall to an extravascular site three days post-injection. Pore diameters in the basal lamina are 0.54 μm (left) and 0.41 μm (right) [108].

Next, tumor cell organelles such as glycogen granules and rough endoplasmic reticulum membranes move into this balloon-like protrusion, followed by large organelles such as mitochondria and the Golgi complex. As a result of cytoplasmic streaming, the cell mass is transferred progressively across the basement membrane so that eventually the entire cell comes to reside in the extravascular location. In all examples of this phenomenon examined by serial or semi-serial sections, the pores made by tumor cells in the basement membrane were very small (diameter 0.07–1.80 μm) and were confined to the sites of tumor cell penetration (Figure 31). Similar findings have been reported with other tumor cell types.

B. Segregation-Type Extravasation

Histologic and electron microscopic investigations have shown that certain tumor cell emboli residing in microvessels are covered or completely enclosed by endothelial cells. In this location, tumor cells are segregated from the fluid phase of the bloodstream without undergoing complete extravasation into perivascular tissues. Two different segregation patterns have been observed. One involves the development of septum-like endothelial cells within a capillary, which cover the tumor cell embolus and lead to complete occlusion of the capillary. This type of segregation has been observed in three-day-old AH7974 tumors growing in the brain (Figure 32).

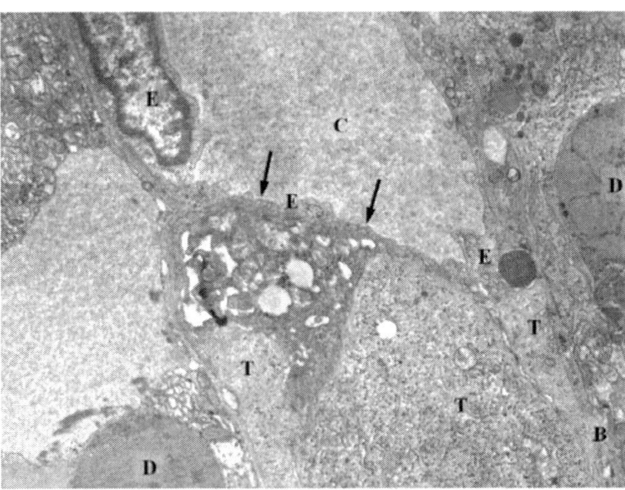

Figure 32. Tumor cells (T) are segregated from the bloodstream (arrows) by endothelial cells (E). B: vascular basement membrane. C: capillary lumen. D: perivascular dense body [108].

In the second type of segregation, tumor cells lodged in capillaries or small veins are also covered or enclosed by endothelial cells, but the vascular lumen remains partially open. This latter process has been described in a diversity of tumors in different organ vascular beds, such as AH13 hepatoma in the adrenal gland, AH7974F hepatoma in the liver, AH7974 hepatoma in the brain, Morris hepatoma in the lung, and L2C leukemia cells in the liver.

C. Explosion-Type Extravasation

A more dramatic form of extravasation has been identified in AH7974 hepatoma cells arrested in the kidney. In eight-day-old tumors, a large number of tumor cells were found in Bowman's space leading to ischemia and atrophy of the glomerular capillary tuft. The remainder of the tuft was filled with proliferating tumor cells, and it expanded like a ball.

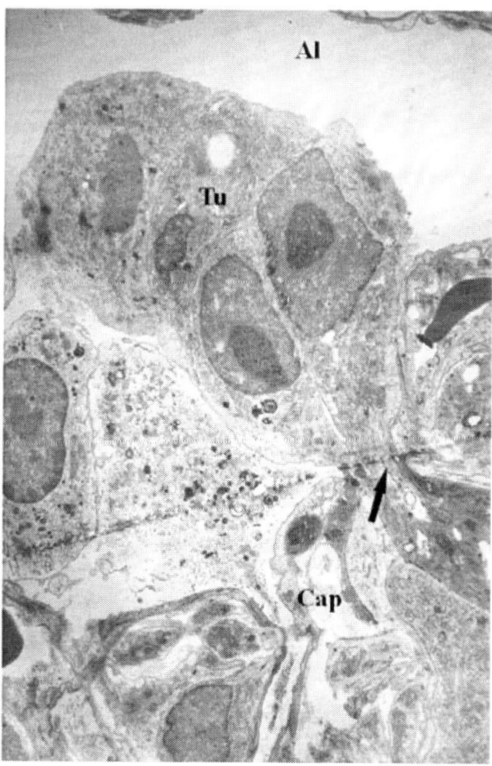

Figure 33. An aggregation of AH601 tumor cells (Tu) flowing out (arrow) explosively from the capillary (Cap) to the alveolar sac (Al) through a split in the vessel wall (arrow). The tumor mass is strangulated and elongated at the split [107].

In regions adjacent to the tumor cells, the endothelial cells were absent, exposing the underlying basement membrane. The outer layer of the basement membrane of the glomerulus was usually thin but did not show any evidence of rupture. Examination of serial sections of this area revealed that the tuft, which was swollen like a ball with tumor cells, contained discrete circular lesions in the basement membrane that were not observed in deeper sections or elsewhere. We consider that aggregated tumor cells had emigrated through the structural defect in the basement membrane created by this lesion [35, 107].

A similar example was identified in rat lung with a seven-day-old AH601 tumor in which an aggressive tumor cell mass appeared to be strangulated at the point where the vessel was ruptured (Figure 33). This is analogous to the renal tumor discussed above. Although it is, of course, impossible to define the kinetics of extravasation from static morphologic measurements, the ultrastructural appearance of these lesions is suggestive of a rapid "herniation" of tumor emboli. We speculate that this process probably involves a rapid, explosive, and forced expulsion of tumor cells through the defect in the vessel wall. Despite extensive analysis of large numbers of tissue sections, only the two examples cited above have been identified in which a defect in the basement membrane can be reliably recognized. No previous reports of similar lesions have been found in the literature.

D. Others

The following was observed when rat ascites hepatoma AH7974 cells in the brain, which were injected via the carotid artery three days before, were investigated by electron microscopy. Although fundamentally this could be categorized as segregation-type extravasation, we have classified it "others." This is a case where a tumor cell was found in the cerebral cortex without surrounding blood vessel structures; we believe the reason why blood vessel structures disappear around the tumor cells is because there is not enough time for the tumor cell to have migrated from the blood vessel. We have never observed this situation and can find no such report; hence, we have doubted its likelihood for a long time. Nevertheless, Hori et al. [127] recently reported a microcinematographic study supporting the possibility of this process occurring (Figure 34). Because it is difficult to define the blood vessel wall basement membrane by the method they employed, further investigations are required.

The above description is of hematogenous metastasis. We do not know how tumor cells achieve extravasation in lymphatic metastasis, but it appears that the extravasation mode is different from that in hematogenous metastasis.

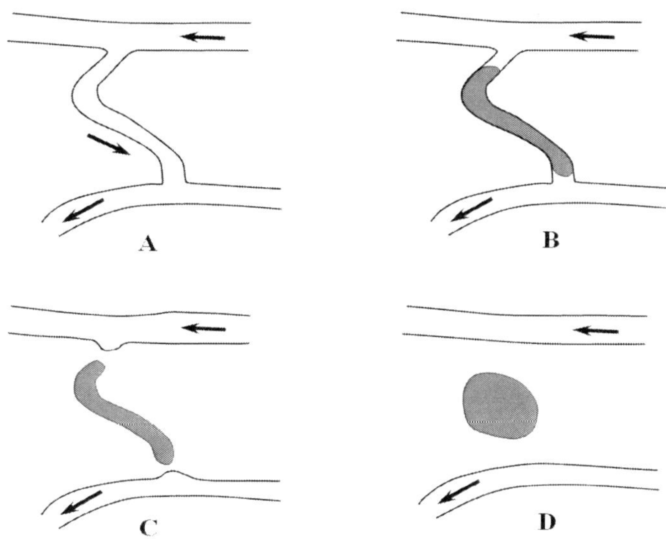

Figure 34. Schematic representation of extravasation of tumor cells. Circulating tumor cells embolize and lodge in a blood capillary (A, B). When the capillary becomes stenotic, the capillary wall disappears resulting in extravasation of the tumor cells (C, D) [127] (with permission of first author).

Tumor cells are likely to proliferate within lymphatic vessels and within marginal sinuses of lymph nodes. Using transmission electron microscopy, we investigated the mode of tumor cell migration from the abdominal cavity to previously injured peritoneal tissues [38]. It was found that tumor cells were attached to regenerative mesothelial cells or the exposed submesothelial basal lamina using their microvilli or cytoplasmic processes and were then enclosed or covered by elongated cytoplasmic protrusions of mesothelial cells. The cytoplasmic processes of the tumor cells breached those of the mesothelial cells and eventually the basal lamina, resulting in further migration of tumor cells into the submesothelial granulation tissue, where they proliferated to form tumor nodules.

5.3. Factors Affecting the Extravasation of Tumor Cells

We consider two types of tumor cell extravasation, active and passive, as similar for tumor cell intravasation. The active type is related to the invasion capacity of tumor cells, whereas the passive one is related to the regenerative activity of vascular endothelial cells and mesothelial cells.

A. Invasive Potential of Tumor Cells

A.1. Target Site of Endothelial Cell Lining

Rarely do almost all tumor cells, including those of hematopoietic origin, migrate through the intercellular junctions of vascular endothelial cells during extravasation. Rather, they migrate through the endothelial cell body; some tumor cells utilize the so-called fenestration of endothelial cells for their extravasation. Furthermore, it is possible that the cytoplasmic protrusions of tumor cells invaginate to form pinocytotic vesicles, coated vesicles (pits), and/or caveolae, followed by their deep progression, resulting in the passing of these vesicles through the endothelium of blood vessels. Pinocytotic vesicles transport blood plasma, which contains various substances necessary for cellular metabolism. Coated vesicles and caveolae contain clathrin and caveolin, respectively, and are related to the absorption of lipids for cell membrane synthesis [128]. As proposed by Dvorak et al. [129], the vesiculo–vacuolar organelle (VVO) in the microvasculature may be a possible route of tumor cell extravasation. Since these transport systems rigidly select the substances transported, it is reasonable to consider that metastatic tumor cells possess cell membrane component(s) having function(s) corresponding to endothelial cell function.

A.2. Invadopodia and Basement Membrane Degradation Enzymes Involved in Extravasation

The development of tumor cell invadopodia (cytoplasmic projections, protrusions, and pseudopodia) is crucial not only during the active form of tumor cell extravasation but also during any stage of the metastatic process as previously described. We believe that the invadopodia is a destructive “weapon” of metastatic tumor cells for destruction of surrounding tissues.

As described before, Gonda et al. [95] demonstrated that membrane fluidity increases during intravasation, peaks in blood vessels, decreases during extravasation, and is higher in locally formed pseudopodia (invadopodia). Albiges-Rizo et al. [130] described how invadopodia, located at the cell–matrix adhesion site, are correlated with the presence of dynamic, actin-rich membrane structures, and the involvement of Rho GTPase Cdc42 in inducing invadopodial-membrane protrusion. Currently, we can image the trafficking, accumulation, and release of certain types of matrix proteases such as MT1-MMP in the invadopodia of the tumor cells at the invasion front [131] (see Figures 31, 35). However, further studies are required to elucidate the factor(s) inducing the formation and extension of tumor cell invadopodia and the cell membrane characteristics of invadopodia.

A.3. Cytoplasmic Streaming of Metastatic Tumor Cells

In addition to enzymatic modification of host tissue barriers by tumor cells, the deformability of tumor cells is also considered to be an important factor facilitating tumor cell extravasation. Sato et al. [88] demonstrated that when tumor cells were passed through small pores of <5 μm diameter, they necessarily underwent significant degeneration and necrosis. However, we have observed that tumor cells are sometimes capable of passing through pores of that size. Therefore, we believe that there is another possible mechanism by which viable tumor cells are able to pass through pores of <5 μm diameter. The cytoplasmic streaming of tumor cells, as shown in Figure 31, is a mechanism by which tumor cells can pass through very small pores of even <2 μm diameter without any cellular damage. Unfortunately, no detailed studies have been carried out on the rheological and other mechanical properties of tumor cells that may influence their ability to form pseudopodia and other surface extensions. We observed that metastatic tumor cells rapidly lose their microvilli after their arrest in capillaries, leaving a smooth surface that is subsequently modified by the formation of pseudopodia [21, 108]. In the case of AH7974 cells lodged in cerebral capillaries, the surface microvilli were lost two days after metastatic cell arrest. Distinct tumor cell pseudopodia were first detected three days after arrest, at which time tumor cell extravasation began. A similar sequence of cell surface changes has been detected in morphometric analyses of Yoshida sarcoma cells arrested in liver sinusoids [132].

A.4. Carbohydrate-Selectin/Integrin Interaction in Lodgement and Extravasation of Tumor Cells

Although there is little information on the molecular mechanisms involved in tumor cell lodgement followed by extravasation, several researchers have described tumor cell extravasation occurring in a manner similar to the process of leukocyte extravasation. The rolling mediated by cytokine-activated endothelial selectins is followed by firmer adhesions with β1 and β2 integrin subunits to an activated endothelium and subsequent diapedesis, which most likely involves activation of Rho GTPases, which are regulators of cytoskeletal rearrangement and motility. Among these reports, of particular interest is the report that states that there is evidence that binding of MUC1, a transmembrane immunoglobulin protein with a large extracellular mucin domain, to endothelial ICAM promotes transendothelial migration (TEM) of tumor cells [133]. As described in latter section (Chapter III, Section 3), we propose that expression of aberrant MUC1 protein with Tn antigen by human breast cancer cells is related to lymphatic metastasis [71]. We also proposed different combinations of selectin ligands in hematogenous liver metastasis and lymph node metastasis of colorectal cancer; expression of sialyl-Lewis^a and sialyl-Lewis^x antigen in the former and expression of galactose (Gal)/*N*-acethyl-galactosamine (GalNAc) antigen in the latter [134], although we did not know whether extravasation of tumor cells is mediated by such carbohydrates.

B. Factors Affecting Passive Extravasation

Newly elongated vascular endothelial cells bring about passive extravasation through the disruption of the vascular lumen and disappearance of the vascular walls in which tumor cells lodge (Figures 32, 35).

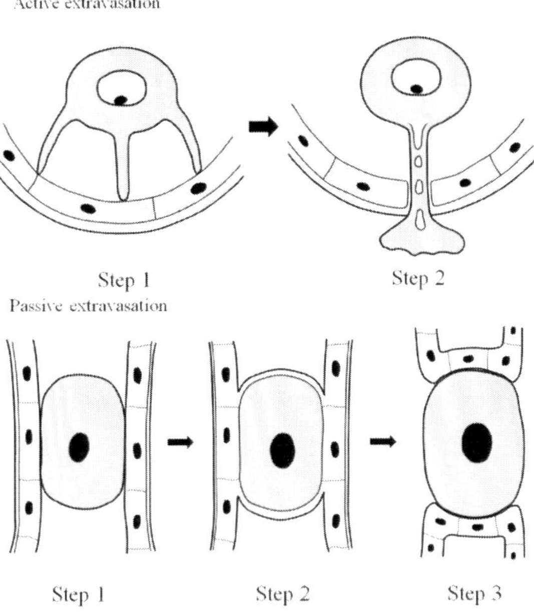

Figure 35. Schematic presentation of the two types of tumor cell extravasation. There are two types of extravasation, active and passive. Active type of tumor cell extravasation involves tumor cell adhesion (Step 1), followed by its transmigration through the endothelial cell body and basement membrane (Step 2). On the other hand, in passive extravasation, some tumor cells arrested in blood vessels (Step 1) are covered by elongated endothelial cells accompanied by basement membrane (Step 2), which then disappear (Step 3), resulting in tumor cell extravasation.

We believe that the disruption of the vascular lumen by newly elongated endothelial cells occurs not only in tumor cells but also during thrombus formation, suggesting that this phenomenon may be a useful method of elimination of foreign bodies. We do not know the mechanisms of disappearance of vascular components that surround lodged tumor cells, but it is likely that the endothelial cells undergo ischemic degeneration. Although vascular basement membrane degradation by tumor cells is likely to occur, another form of basement membrane degradation may be possible, such as basal lamina type IV collagen degradation observed during hemorrhagic transformation following human ischemic stroke [135].

6. Metastatic Foci

6.1. Fate of Extravasated Tumor Cells

Tumor cell extravasation is a prerequisite for metastasis formation, but this does not imply establishment of metastasis. After extravasation, there are approximately five possible courses that tumor cells pursue (Table 4, Figure 36). In course 1, tumor cells die. In course 2, tumor cells migrate to the appropriate tissue where these cells proliferate (Figure 36). In course 3, tumor cells proliferate at the tissues (early growth) where these cells extravasate, followed by metastatic growth.

In course 4, metastatic tumor cells further metastasize to other tissues. In course 5, tumor cells in courses 2, 3 and 4 become dormant. Here, "proliferation" implies that tumor cells proliferate to form a tumor of 2–3 mm in size, a process being called early growth. In this meaning, "growth" implies that tumor cells form a tumor more than 2–3 mm in size.

As suggested by several experimental studies including ours, extravasated tumor cells require fertile soil to begin proliferation [136]. We consider that the tissue at which tumor extravasation occurs is likely to be injured and that such a tissue in combination with repair tissue provides fertile environment for tumor cells to proliferate.

We [14] termed this concept the "microinjury hypothesis." This concept will be described in detail in Chapter II, but we would like to state here that tumor growth is facilitated by injured tissue and repaired tissue, such as granulation tissue, by releasing several types of growth factors related to tissue regeneration and abundant vascular networks [137, 138]: EGF, TGF, HGF

(SF), FGF, PDGF, and IGFs, all of which are involved in tissue injury and granulation.

Table 4. Fate of extravasated tumor cells

Course 1.	Tumor cells die.
Course 2.	Tumor cells migrate to another tissue (postextravasation movement), proliferate, and grow wherein tumor cells form metastatic foci.
Course 3.	Tumor cells proliferate in the tissue in which the tumor cells extravasate and then metastasize.
Course 4.	Metastatic tumor cells further metastasize to other tissues.
Course 5.	Tumor cells in courses 2, 3, and 4 become dormant.

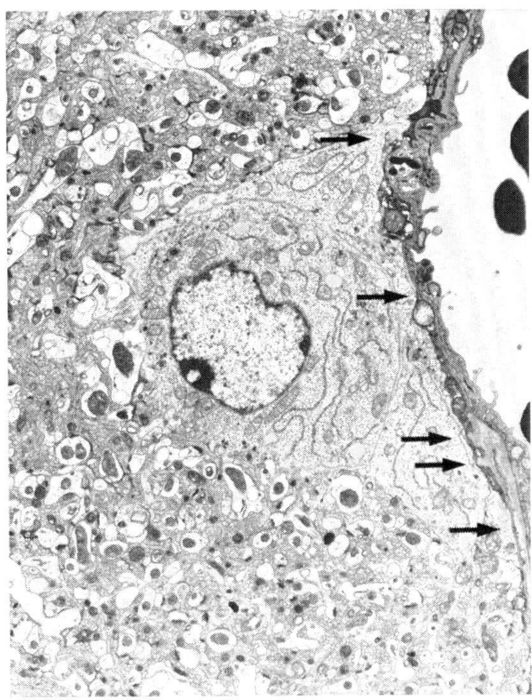

Figure 36. Migration of a B16-B14b tumor cell (T) to the cerebral vein (V). A large part of the tumor cell cytoplasm is attached to perivascular astrocytes and a small part to the basal lamina (arrow). The B16-B14b cell is a variant subline, which was selected in vivo for enhanced brain surface colonization in C57BL/6 mice. The extravasated tumor cells appear to migrate around a large blood vessel in brain meninges [36] [105].

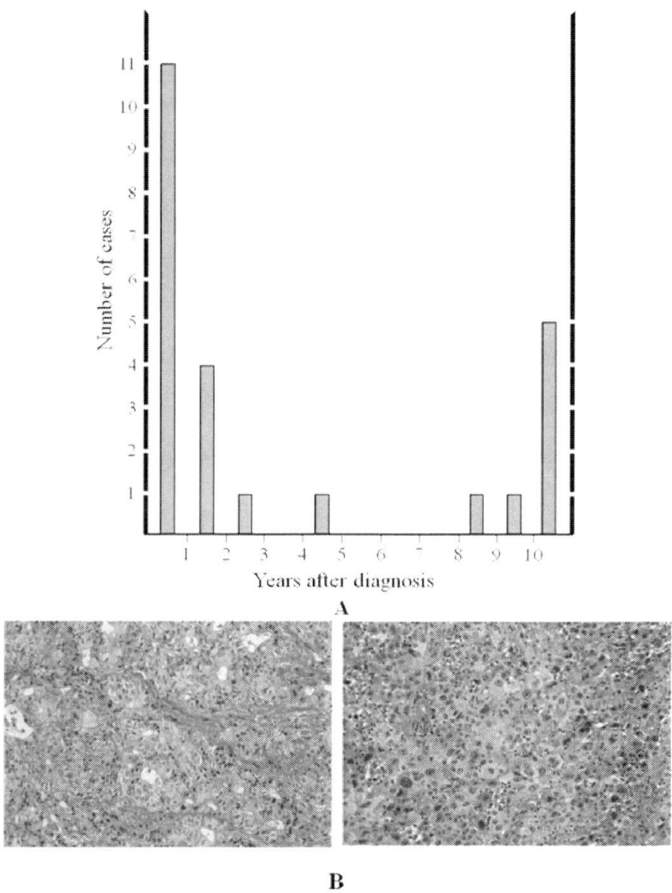

Figure 38. Prognosis of thyroid cancer patients after surgery. A: There appear two types of recurrence between surgery and death caused by metastatic recurrence: relatively early recurrences until five years after surgery and late recurrence eight years after surgery. B: The picture of papillary carcinoma on the left side was obtained from surgery specimen, and the metastatic recurrent tumor was anaplastic carcinoma, as shown on right side [Kawaguchi T, unpublished data].

6.3. Contribution of Pathology for Metastatic Tumors

For a long time, it has been believed that metastasis indicates the most advanced stage of a malignant tumor and that patients with metastasis are incurable by therapy. However, recent advances in diagnosis and therapy for metastatic tumors have offered the possibility of a cure in some patients with metastasis.

Table 5. List of antibodies used

Antibody	Application
AE1/AE3	Epithelial tumor
AFP (α-fetoprotein)	Germ cell tumor, hepatocellular carcinoma
ALK	Lymphoma/leukemia
AMACR (α-methylacyl-CoA racemase)	Prostatic carcinoma
bcl-2	Lymphoma/leukemia
Cadherin	Lobular carcinoma (breast)
Calponin	Smooth muscle tumor
Calretinin	Mesothelioma
CA19-9	Pancreatic cancer, gastric cancer
CD3	Lymphoma/leukemia
CD4	Lymphoma/leukemia
CD5	Lymphoma/leukemia
CD8	Lymphoma/leukemia
CD10	Lymphoma/leukemia, endometrial stromal tumor
CD20	Lymphoma/leukemia
CD23	Lymphoma/leukemia
CD30	Lymphoma/leukemia
CD31	Angiosarcoma
CD34	Gastrointestinal stromal tumor (GIST)
CD45 (LCA)	Lymphoma/leukemia
CD45RO (UCHL)	Lymphoma/leukemia
CD56	Neuroendocrine tumor
CD68 (kp-1)	Macrophage/monocytic tumor
CD79α	B cell lymphoma, plasmacytoma
CD99	Ewing sarcoma、synovial sarcoma
CD138	Plasmcytoma, multiple myeloma
CDX2	Intestinal carcinoma
CEA (Carcinoembryonic antigen)	Gasrointestinal carcinoma
Chromogranin	Neuroendocrine tumor
c-kit (CD117)	GIST
CK5/6	Mesothelioma
CK10/13	Squamous cell carcinoma
CK7	Various carcinomas
CK14	Squamous cell carcinoma (lung)
CK17	Squamous cell carcinoma
CK19	Cholangiocarcinoma
CK20	Various carcinomas
CyclinD1	Lymphom/leukemia
34βE12	Squamous cell carcinoma
Desmin	Myosarcoma
D2-40	Lymphangiosarcoma, mesothelioma
DOG-1	GIST
E-cadherin	Breast cancer

Antibody	Application
EMA (epithelial membrane antigen)	Mesothelioma, meningioma
ER (estrogen receptor)	Breast cancer, endometrial cancer
Estradiol	Ovarian tumor
GFAP (glial fibrillary acidic acid)	Glioma tumor, glioblastoma
Gastric mucin	Gastric cancer
hCG (human chorionic gonadotropin)	Choriocarcinoma
HER2/neu (c-erbB-2 oncoprotein)	Breast cancer, gastric cancer
HMB45	Malignant melanoma
hPL (human placenta lactogen)	Placenta site trophoblastic tumor
IgA, D, G, M	Myeloma
Insulin	Insulinoma
Manmmaglobin	Breast cancer
Melan-A	Melanoma
MPO	Leukemia
MUC-1	Breast cancer, pancreatic cancer
MUC-2	Colorectal cancer
MUC-5AC	Gastric cancer
MUC-6	Gastric cancer
Myogenin	Skeletal muscle
Napsin A	Lung cancer (adenocarcinoma)
PgR (Progesterone receptor)	Breast cancer, endometrial cancer
PLAP (placental alkaline phosphatase)	Dysgerminoma, germinoma
PSA (prostate-specific antigen)	Prostatic cancer
SMA (smooth muscle actin)	Smooth muscle tumor
Synaptophysin	Neuroendocrine carcinoma
S100	Neurogenic tumor, liposarcoma
TdT (terminal deoxynucleotidyl transferase)	Lymphoma
Thyroglobulin	Thyroid cancer
TTF-1 (thyroid transcription factor-1)	Thyroid cancer, lung cancer (adenocarcinoma)
Uroplakin	Urinary bladder cancer
Vimentin	Mesenchymal tumor
WT1	Wilms tumor
κ light chain	Myeloma
λ light chain	Myeloma
gpIIb/IIIa	Leukemia

Pathology has contributed to recent advances, particularly from the viewpoint of identification of the primary tumor. Pathologists are able to identify the primary tumor of metastatic tumors by histopathological and immunohistochemical examinations. Table 5 shows our list of antibodies used for immunohistochemistry.

References

[1] Berenblum, I. The nature of tumour growth. In: Florey L, editor. *General Pathology*. London: Lloyd-Luke; 1970; 645-667.

[2] Willis, RA. *Pathology of tumors*, Fourth edition. London: Butterworths; 1967.

[3] Willis, RA. *The Spread of Tumours in the Human Body*, Third Edition. London: Buuterworths; 1973.

[4] Weiss, L. The pathophysiology of metastasis within the lymphatic system. In: Weiss L, Gilbert HA, Ballon SC, editors. *Lymphatic System Metastais*. Boston: GK Hall Medical Publisher; 1980; 2-40.

[5] Kihara, T. Das extravaskulaere Saftbahnsystem. *Okajimas Fol. Anat. Jpn.*, 1956, *28*, 601-621.

[6] Takubo, K; Nishimura, H; Taniguchi, Y; Sasajima, K; Nakagawa, H; Miyamoto, H; Fujita, K. Junctions between intraepithelial carcinoma and non-neoplastic tissue of the esophagus. Light and electron microscopic studies. *Acta. Pathol. Jpn.*, 1984, 34, 785-796.

[7] Dingemans, KP; Mooi, WJ. Invasion of lung tissue by bronchogenic squamous-cell carcinomas: interaction of tumor cells and lung parenchyma in the tumor periphery. *Int. J. Cancer*, 1986, 37, 11-19.

[8] Sugino, T; Kawaguchi, T; Suzuki, T. Sequential process of blood-borne lung metastases of spontaneous mammary carcinoma in C3H mice. *Int. J. Cancer*, 1993, 55, 141-147.

[9] Odashima, S. Establishment of ascites hepatomas in the rat, 1951-1962. *J. Natl. Cancer Inst. Monogr.*, 1964, 16, 51-93.

[10] Coman, DR. Mechanisms responsible for the origin and distribution of blood-borne tumor metastases: a review. *Cancer Res.*, 1953, 13, 397-404.

[11] Takeichi, M. Cadherin cell adhesion receptors as a morphogenetic regulator. *Science*, 1991, 251, 1451-1455.

[12] Hayashi, H; Ishimaru, Y. Morphological and biochemical aspects of adhesiveness and dissociation of cancer cells. *Int. Rev. Cytol.*, 1981, 70, 139-215.

[13] Nabeshima, K; Inoue, T; Shimao, Y; Okada, Y; Itoh, Y; Seiki, M; Koono, M. Front-cell-specific expression of membrane-type 1 matrix metalloproteinase and gelatinase A during cohort migration of colon carcinoma cells induced by hepatocyte growth factor/scatter factor. *Cancer Res.*, 2000, 60, 3364-3369.

[14] Kawaguchi, T; Nakamura, K. Relationship between transcerebral

passage of tumor cells and brain metastasis. *Gann.*, 1977, 68, 65-71.

[15] Bosman, FT; Havenith, MG; Visser, R; Cleutjens, JP. Basement membranes in neoplasia. *Prog. Histochem. Cytochem.*, 1992, 24, 1992, 1–92.

[16] Barsky, SH; Siegal, GP; Jannotta, F; Liotta, LA. Loss of basement membrane components by invasive tumors but not by their benign counterparts. *Lab. Invest.*, 1983, 49, 140-147.

[17] Liotta, LA; Tryggvason, K; Garbisa, S; Hart, I; Foltz, CM; Shafie, S. Metastatic potential correlates with enzymatic degradation of basement membrane collagen. *Nature*, 1980, 284, 67-68.

[18] Nakajima, M; Irimura, T; Di Ferrante, D; Di Ferrante, N; Nicolson, GL. Heparan sulfate degradation: relation to tumor invasive and metastatic properties of mouse B16 melanoma sublines. *Science*, 1983, 220, 611-613.

[19] Wakabayashi, H; Kawaguchi, T. Fibronectin degradation by human gastric carcinoma cell lines and its associated proteases in relation to stromal invasion in nude mice. *Invasion Metastasis*, 1992, 12, 284-300.

[20] Kawaguchi, T; Igarashi, S; Kono, K. Tumor cell adhesiveness and metastasis- its pathological bases. *Biotherapy*, 1993, 7, 1141-1150. (in Japanese).

[21] Kawaguchi, T; Endo, M; Tobai, S; Nakamura, K. Behavior pattern of rat ascites tumor cells arrested in liver sinusoids: an electron microscopic study. *Gann.*, 1979, 70, 277-290.

[22] Liotta, LA. Tumor invasion and metastasis- role of the extracellular matrix: Rhoads Memorial Award Lecture. *Cancer Res.*, 1986, 46, 1-7.

[23] Ooishi, M; Kawaguchi, T; Hoshi, K; Morimura, Y; Sato, A; Suzuki, T. Immunohistochemical demonstration of laminin in endometrial cancer of uterus in relation to its invasion and metastasis. *Acta Obst. Gynec. Jpn.*, 1995, 47, 955-956. (in Japanese).

[24] Pauli, BU. Host tissue resistance to tumor invasion. In: Mareel MM, Calman KC, editors. *Invasion: experimental and clinical implications*. Oxford Univ. Press; 1985; 205-227.

[25] Ono, M; Sakamoto, M; Ino, Y; Moriya, Y; Sugihara, K; Muto, T; Hirohashi, S. Cancer cell morphology at the invasive front and expression of cell adhesion-related carbohydrate in the primary lesion of patients with colorectal carcinoma with liver metastasis. *Cancer*, 1996, 78, 1179-1186.

[26] Sylven, B. Some factors relating to the invasiveness and destructiveness of solid malignant tumours. In: Denoix P, editor. *Mechanisms of*

invasion in cancer UICC Monogr. Series Vol.6. Heidelberg: Springer-Verlag; 1967; 47-60.

[27] Hamada, J; Takeichi, N; Okada, F; Ren, J; Li, X; Hosokawa, M; Kobayashi, H. Progression of weakly malignant clone cells derived from rat mammary carcinoma by host cells reactive to plastic plates. *Jpn. J. Cancer Res.*, 1992, 83, 483-490.

[28] Sakakura, T; Kusano, I. Tenascin in tissue perturbation repair. *Acta Pathol. Jpn.*,1991, 41, 247-258.

[29] Nakahara, W; Fukuoka, F. Toxohormone: a characteristic toxic substance produced by cancer tissue. *Gann*, 1949, 40, 45-71.

[30] Brandes, D; Anton, E; Schofield, B. Invasion of skeletal and smooth muscle by L1210 leukemia. *Cancer Res.*, 1967, 27, 2159-2178.

[31] Galasko, CS; Muckle, DS. Intrasarcolemmal proliferation of the VX2 carcinoma. *Br. J. Cancer*, 1974, 29, 59-65.

[32] Gabbert, H; Gerharz, CD; Ramp, U; Bohl, J. The nature of host tissue destruction in tumor invasion. An experimental investigation on carcinoma and sarcoma xenotransplants. *Virchows Arch. B Cell Pathol. Incl. Mol. Pathol.*, 1987, 52, 513-527.

[33] Igarashi, S; Kawaguchi, T. Ultrastructure of invasion of the adult rat hepatocyte monolayer by rat ascites hepatoma variant sublines. *Invasion Metastasis*, 1993, 13, 132-146.

[34] Katsuta, H; Takaoka, T; Nagai, Y. Interaction in culture between normal and tumor cells of rats. In: Katsuta H, editor. *Cancer cells in culture*. Tokyo: University of Tokyo Press; 1968; 157-168.

[35] Nakamura, K; Kawaguchi, T; Asahina, S; Sakurai, T; Ebina, Y; Yokoya, S; Morita, M. Electronmicroscopic studies on extravasation of tumor cells and early foci of hematogenous metastases. *Gann Mongr. Cancer Res.*, 1977, 20, 57-71.

[36] Kawaguchi, T; Kawaguchi, M; Dulski, KM; Nicolson, GL. Cellular behavior of metastatic B16 melanoma in experimental blood-borne implantation and cerebral invasion: an electron microscopic study. *Invasion Metastasis*, 1985, 5, 16-30.

[37] Kawaguchi, T; Nakamura, K. Analysis of the lodgement and extravasation of tumor cells in experimental models of hematogenous metastasis. *Cancer Metastasis Rev.*, 1986, 5, 77-94.

[38] Nakashima, Y; Kawaguchi, T; Nakamura, K. The mechanisms of metastasis formation in injured parietal peritoneum by Yoshida sarcoma cells: an electron microscopic study. *Fukushima J. Med. Sci.*, 1985, 31, 17-28.

[39] Kerbel, RS; Lagarde, AE; Dennis, JW; Nestel, FP; Donaghue, TP; Siminovitch, L; Fulchignoni-Lataud, MC. Relevance of spontaneous in vivo tumor-host cell fusion to tumor progression and metastasis evaluated using a series of lectin-resistant mutant tumor sublines. In: Nicolson GL, Milas L, editors. *Cancer invasion and metastasis: biologic and therapeutic aspects*. New York: Raven Press; 1984; 47-79.

[40] Takahashi, T; Ishikura, H; Motohara, T; Okushiba, S; Dohke, M; Katoh, H. Perineural invasion by ductal adenocarcinoma of the pancreas. *J. Surg. Oncol.*, 1997, 65, 164-170.

[41] Shirai, K; Ebata, T; Oda, K; Nishio, H; Nagasaka, T; Nimura, Y; Nagino, M. Perineural invasion is a prognostic factor in intrahepatic cholangiocarcinoma. *World J. Surg.*, 2008, 32, 2395-2402.

[42] Larson, DL; Rodin, AE; Roberts, DK; Osteen, WK; Rapperport, AS; Lewis, SR. Perineural lymphatics: Myth or Fact. *Am. J. Surg.*, 1966, 112, 488-492.

[43] Pister, PWT; Kelsen, DP; Powell, SM; Tepper, JE. Cancer of the stomach. In: DeVita VT, Jr, Hellman S, Rosenberg SA, editors. *Cancer: Principles and Practice of Oncology, 7th edition*. Philadelphia: Lippincott Williams and Wilkins; 2005; 909-944.

[44] Mosely, JM; Dickson, DR. Vascular invasion in lung cancer. Clinical-pathologic significance. *Am. Rev. Respir. Dis.*, 1960, 82, 807-809.

[45] Warren, BA; Marchalonis, JJ; Hanna, MG; Fidler, IJ; editors. Origin and fate of blood-borne tumor emboli. In: *Cancer Biology Reviews vol. 2*. New York: Dekker; 1981; 95-169.

[46] Kung, PC; Lee, JC; Bakay, L. Vascular invasion by glioma cells in man: an electron microscopic study. *J. Neurosurg.*,1969, 31, 339-345.

[47] Kawaguchi, T; Igarashi, S; Sugino, T; Fukui, K; Nakamura, K. The mechanisms of cancer metastasis; an electron microscopic study. *Nihon Rinsho*, 1987, 45, 237-249. (in Japanese).

[48] Bruyn, PPH; Cho, Y; Michelson, S. Endothelial attachment and plasmalemmal apposition in the transcellular movement of intravascular leukemic cells entering the myeloid parenchyma. *Am. J. Anatomy*, 1989, 186, 115-126.

[49] Azzarelli, B; Mirkin, LD; Goheen, M; Muller, J; Crockett, C. The leptomeningeal vein. A site of re-entry of leukemic cells into the systemic circulation. *Cancer*, 1984, 54, 1333-1343.

[50] Constantinides, P; Hewitt, D; Harkey, M. Vessel invasion by tumor cells an ultrastructural study. *Virchows. Archiv. A. Pathol. Anat.*, 1989, 415, 335-346.

[51] Sugino, T; Kawaguchi, T; Suzuki, T. Sequential process of blood-borne lung metastases of spontaneous mammary carcinoma in C3H mice. *Int. J. Cancer*, 1993, 55, 141-147.

[52] Sugino, T; Kusakabe, T; Hoshi, N; Yamaguchi, T; Kawaguchi, T; Goodison, S; Sekimata, M; Homma, Y; Suzuki. T. An invasion-independent pathway of blood-borne metastasis: a new murine mammary tumor model. *Am. J. Pathol.*, 2002, 160, 1973-1980.

[53] Kawaguchi, T. Cancer metastasis: characterization and identification of the behavior of metastatic tumor cells and the cell adhesion molecules, including carbohydrates. *Current Drug Targets- Cardiovasc. Hematol. Dis.*, 2005, 5, 39-64.

[54] Takasawa, H. Experimental lymphatic metastasis. Electron microscopic observation on lymphatic vessel invasion of transplanted tumor cell in rat. *Proc. Jap. Cancer Assoc.*, 1972, 31, 296. (in Japanese).

[55] Araki, K. An ultrastructural evaluation of experimentally induced cancer cell invasion into the lymphatic vessel in rats. *Bull. Osaka Med. Sch.*, 1982, 28, 7-13.

[56] Deutsch, A; Lubach, D; Nissen, S; Neukam, D. Ultrastrucural studies on the invasion of melanomas in initial lymphatics of human skin. *J. Invest. Dermal.*, 1992, 98, 64-67.

[57] Carr, I; McGinty, F; Norris, P. The fine structure of neoplastic invasion: invasion of liver, skeletal muscle and lymphatic vessels by the Rd/3 tumour. *J. Pathol.*, 1976, 118, 91-99.

[58] Paku, S; Paweletz, N; Spiess, E; Aulenbacher, P; Werling, H-O; Knierim, M. Ultrastructural analysis of experimentally induced invasion in the rat lung by tumor cells metastasizing lymphatically. *Anticancer Res.*,1986, 6, 957-966.

[59] Tobai, S; Kawaguchi, T; Asahina, S; Nakamura, K. Some findings on the intravasation of Yoshida sarcoma cells in the omentum. *Gann*, 1980, 71, 578-579.

[60] Hagiwara, A; Takahashi, T; Sawai, K; Taniguchi, H; Shimotsuma, M; Okano, S; Sakakura, C; Tsujimoto, H; Osaki, K; Sasaki, K; Sasaki, S; Shirasu, M. Milky spots as the implantation site for malignant cells in peritoneal dissemination in mice. *Cancer Res.*, 1993, 53, 1993, 687-692.

[61] Takemori, N; Hirai, K; Onodera, R; Saito, N; Namiki, M. Light and electron microscopic study of omental milky spots in New Zealand Black mice, with special reference to the extramedullary hematopoiesis. *Anat. Embryol.*, 1994, 189, 215-226.

[62] Azzali, G. Tumor cell transendothelial passage in the absorbing

lymphatic vessel of transgenic adenocarcinoma mouse prostate. *Am. J. Pathol.*, 2007, 170, 334-346.

[63] Kobayashi, T; Asahina, S; Tobai, S; Kitamura, H; Nakamura, K. An experimental study on the growth of ascites hepatoma AH-130 inoculated in the rectal abdominal muscle into the peritoneal cavity. *Fukushima Igaku Zasshi*, 1979, 29, 145-157. (in Japanese).

[64] Sugino T, Yamaguchi T, Hoshi N, Kusakabe T, Ogura G, Goodison S, Suzuki T. Sinusoidal tumor angiogenesis is a key component in hepatocellular carcinoma metastasis. *Clin. Exp. Metastasis* , 2008, 25, 835-841.

[65] Nakanishi, H; Takenaga, K; Oguri, K; Yoshida, A; Okayama, M. Morphological characteristics of tumors formed by Lewis lung carcinoma-derived cloned cell lines with different metastatic potentials; structural differences in their basement membranes formed in vivo. *Virchow Arch A Pathol. Anat. Histopathol.*, 1987, 411, 223-232.

[66] Wyckoff, JB; Jones, JG; Condeelis, JS; Segall, JE. A critical step in metastasis: *in vitro* analysis of intravasation at the primary tumor. *Cancer Res.*, 2000, 60, 2504-2511.

[67] Dua, RS; Gui, GPH; Isacke, CM. Endothelial adhesion molecules in breast cancer invasion into the vascular and lymphatic systems. *Eur. J. Surg. Oncol.*, 2005, 31, 824-832.

[68] Makrilia, N; Kollias, A; Manolopoulos, L; Syrigos, K. Cell adhesion molecules: role and clinical significance in cancer. *Cancer Invest.*, 2009, 27, 1023-1037.

[69] Kawaguchi, T; Takazawa, H; Imai, S; Morimoto, J; Watanabe, T. Lack of polymorphism in MUC1 tandem repeats in cancer cells is related to breast cancer progression in Japanese woman. *Breast Cancer Res. Treat.*, 2005, 92, 223-230.

[70] Suzuki, O; Nozawa, Y; Kawaguchi, T; Abe, M. α-2, 6-sialylation of L-PHA reactive oligosaccharides and expression of N-acetylglucosaminyltransferase V in human diffuse large B cell lymphoma. *Oncol. Rep.*, 2003, 10, 1759-1764.

[71] Kawaguchi, T; Takazawa, H; Imai, S; Morimoto, J; Watanabe, T; Kanno, M; Igarashi, S. Expression of Vicia villosa agglutinin (VVA)-binding glycoprotein in primary breast cancer cells in relation to lymphatic metastasis: is atypical MUC1 bearing Tn antigen receptor of VVA? *Breast Cancer Res. Treat.*, 2006, 98, 31-43.

[72] Kawaguchi, T; Imai, S; Haga, S; Morimoto, J; Honda, T. Demonstration and partial identification of aberrant Muc1 bearing Tn antigen in rat

ascites hepatoma AH109A cells with strong lymph node metastasis propensity. In: Watanabe A, editor. *Cancer Metastasis Research*. New York: Nova Science Publishers; 2008; 147-163.

[73] Kawaguchi, T; Kanno, M; Takazawa, H; Imai, S; Morimoto, J; Haga, S; Honda, T. Lymphatic spreading propensity and aberrant MUC1 bearing TN/TN-like carbohydrate of aggressive breast cancer cells. In: DeFrina RH, editor. *Aggressive Breast Cancer*. New York: Nova Science Publishers; 2009; 199-228.

[74] Kawaguchi, T; Kanno, M; Asahi, S; Honda, T. Relationship between carbohydrate expression profiles of cancer cells and prognosis of breast cancer patients. In: DeFrina RH, editor. *Aggressive Breast Cancer*. New York: Nova Science Publishers; 2009; 231-235.

[75] Rahn, JJ; Shen, Q; Mah, BK; High, JC. MUC1 initiates a calcium signal after ligation by intercellular adhesion molecule-1. *J. Biol. Chem.*, 2004, 279, 29386-29390.

[76] Danussi, C; Coslovi, A; Campa, C; Mucignat, M; Spessotto, P; Uggeri, F; Paoletti, S; Colombatti, A. A newly generated functional antibody identifies Tn antigen as a novel determinant in the cancer cell-lymphatic endothelium interaction. *Glycobiol.*, 2009, 19, 1056-1067.

[77] Azzali, G. The modality of transendothelial passage of lymphocytes and tumor cells in the absorbing lymphatic vessels. *Eur. J. Histochem.*, 2007, 51 suppl. 1, 73-78.

[78] Sugino, T; Yamaguchi, T; Ogura, G; Kusakabe, T; Goodison, S; Homma, Y; Suzuki, T. The secretory leukocyte protease inhibitor (SLPI) suppresses cancer cell invasion but promotes blood-borne metastasis via an invasion-independent pathway. *J. Pathol.*, 2007, 212, 152-160.

[79] Entschladen, F; Drell, TL 4th; Lang, K; Joseph, J; Zaenker, KS. Neurotransmitters and chemokines regulate tumor cell migration: potential for a new pharmacological approach to inhibit invasion and metastasis development. *Curr. Pharm. Des.*, 2005, 11, 403-411.

[80] Müller, A; Homey, B; Soto, H; Ge, N; Catron, D; Buchanan, ME; McClanahan, T; Murphy, E; Yuan, W; Wagner, SN; Barrera, JL; Mohar, A; Verastegui, E; Zlotnik, A. Involvement of chemokine receptors in breast cancer metastasis. *Nature*, 2001, 410, 50-56.

[81] Iwasaki, T. Histological and experimental observations on the destruction of tumor cells in the blood vessels. *J. Pathol. Bacteriol.*, 1915, 20, 85-105.

[82] Fidler, IJ. Metastasis: quantitative analysis of distribution and fate of tumor emboli labeled with 135 I-5-iodo-2-deoxyuridine. *J. Natl. Cancer*

Inst., 1970, 45, 773-782.

[83] Butler, TP; Gullino, PM. Quantitation of cell shedding into efferent blood of mammary adenocarcinoma. *Cancer Res.*, 1975, 35, 512-516.

[84] Koop, S; MacDonald, IC; Luzzi, K; Schmidt, EE; Morris, VL; Gratten, M; Khokha, R; Chambers, AF; Groom, AC. Fate of melanoma cells entering the microcirculation: over 80% survive and extravasate. *Cancer Res.*, 1995, 55, 2520-2523.

[85] Luscher, EF. Serum cytotoxic factors which may influence tumor cell growth. In: *Endogenous Factors Influencing Host Tumor Balance*, Wissler RW et al editors, University Chicago, Chicago, 1967, 167-175.

[86] Glaves, D. Intravascular death of disseminated cancer cells mediated by superoxide anion. *Invasion Metastasis*, 1986, 6, 101-111.

[87] Hanna, N. The role of natural killer cells in the control of tumor growth and metastasis. *Biochim. Biophys. Acta.*, 1985, 780, 213-226.

[88] Sato, H; Suzuki, M. Deformability and viability of tumor cells by transcapillary passage, with reference to organ affinity of metastasis in cancer. In: Weiss L, editor. *Fundamental Aspect of Metastasis*. Amsterdam: North-Holland Publishing; 1976; 311-317.

[89] Weiss, L; Dimitrov, DS; Angelova, M. The hemodynamic destruction of intravascular cancer cells in relation to myocardial metastasis. *Proc. Natl. Acad. Sci. USA*, 1985, 82, 5737-5741.

[90] Kawaguchi, T; Nakamura, K. Survival and experimental metastatic potential of tumor cells circulated *in vitro* under condition of high-speed fluid flow. *Fukushima J. Med. Sci.*, 1987, 33, 47-54.

[91] Simpson, CD. Anoikis resistance and tumor metastasis. *Cancer Lett.*, 2008, 272, 177-185.

[92] Sakuma, Y; Takeuchi, T; Nakamura, Y; Yoshihara, M; Matsukuma, S; Nakayama, H; Ohgane, N; Yokose, T; Kameda, Y; Tsuchiya, E; Miyagi, Y. Lung adenocarcinoma cells floating in lymphatic vessels resist anoikis by expressing phosphorylated Src. *J. Pathol.*, 2010, 220, 574-585.

[93] Raz, A; Ben-Ze'ev, A. Modulation of the metastatic capability in B16 melanoma by cell shape. *Science*, 1983, 221, 1983, 1307-1310.

[94] Folkman, J; Moscona, A. Role of cell shape in growth control. *Nature*, 1978, 273, 345-349.

[95] Gonda, K; Watanabe, TM, Ohuchi N, Higuchi H. In vivo nano-imaging of membrane dynamics in metastatic tumor cells using quantum dots. *J. Biol. Chem.*, 2010, 285, 2750-2757.

[96] Zeidman, I; Buss, JM. Transpulmonary passage of tumor cell emboli.

Cancer Res., 1952, 12, 731-733.

[97] Moore, GE; Sandberg, A; Schubarg, J. Clinical and experimental observation of the occurrence and fate of tumor cells in the blood stream. *Ann. Surg.*, 1957, 146, 580-587.

[98] Nakamura, K; Suzuki, K. Quantitative study on the transpulmonary passage of tumor cells. *Gann*, 1969. 60, 483-497.

[99] Endo, M; Kawaguchi, T; Yokoya, S. Quantitative study on circulating tumor cells in blood, with reference to effect of pretreatment with anticoagulants (I) Evaluation by Conray–Ficoll method. *Fukushima Igaku Zasshi*, 1981, 31, 215-221. (in Japanese)

[100] Wood S, Jr. Pathogenesis of metastasis formation observed *in vivo* in the rabbit ear chamber. *Arch. Pathol.*, 1958, 66, 550-568.

[101] Sato, H; Suzuki, M. Experimental studies on metastasis formation, with special reference to the mechanism of cancer cell lodgement in microcirculation. In: Shimamoto T, Numano F, Addison GM, editors. *Atherogenesis. Vol II, International Congress Series No. 269 (Proc. of the Second International Symposium on Atherogenesis, Thrombogenesis and Pyridinolcarbamate Treatment)*, Amsterdam: Excerpta Medica; 1973; 168-176.

[102] Kawaguchi, T; Endo, M; Yokoya, S; Nakamura, K. Influence of lodgement site on proliferation–kinetics of tumor cells. *Experientia*, 1981, 37, 414-415.

[103] Kawaguchi, T; Endo, M; Yokoya, S; Nakamura, K. Difference in proliferation-kinetics between tumor cells arrested in the brain and liver. *Experientia*, 1982, 38, 1236-1237.

[104] Yokoya, S; Kawaguchi, T; Nakamura, K. Kinetics of lodgement and early proliferation of blood-borne tumor cells (translation for Japanese title). *Nihon Igakkai zasshi*, 1985, 93, 291-293. (in Japanese).

[105] Brunson, KW; Beattie, G; Nicolson, GL. Selection and altered properties of brain-colonising metastatic melanoma. *Nature*, 1978, 272, 543-545.

[106] Irimura, T; Gonzalez, R; Nicolson, GL. Effects of tunicamycin on B16 metastatic melanoma cell surface glycoproteins and blood-borne arrest and survival properties. *Cancer Res.*, 1981, 41, 3411-3418.

[107] Sakurai, T; Ebina, Y; Yokoya, S; Nakamura, K. Electron microscopic studies on extravasation of ascites hepatomas in the kidney and lung. *Fukushima J. Med. Sci.*, 1977, 24, 1-21.

[108] Kawaguchi, T; Tobai, S; Nakamura, K. Extravascular migration of tumor cells in the brain: an electron microscopic study. *Invasion metastasis*, 1982, 2, 40-50.

[109] Warren, BA; Güldner, FH. Ultrastructure of the adhesion of HeLa cells to human vein wall. *Angiologica*, 1969, 6, 32-53.
[110] Warren, BA; Vales, O. The adhesion of thromboplastic tumor emboli to vessel walls in vivo. *Br. J. Exp. Pathol.*, 1972, 53, 301-313.
[111] Cotmore, SF; Carter, RL. Mechanisms of enhanced intrahepatic metastasis in surfactant-treated hamsters: an electron microscopy study. *Int. J. Cancer*, 1973, 11, 725-738.
[112] Sindelar, WF; Tralka, TS; Ketcham, AS. Electron microscopic observations on formation of pulmonary metastases. *J Surg. Res.*, 1975, 18, 137-161.
[113] Eguchi, G; Okada, TS. Ultrastructure of the differentiated cell colony derived from a singly isolated chondrocyte in in vitro culture. *Dev. Growth Differ.*, 1971, 12, 297-312.
[114] Abercrombie, M; Ambrose, EJ. The surface properties of cancer cells: a review. *Cancer Res.*, 1962, 22, 525-548.
[115] Roos, E; Dingemans, KP; van de Pavert, IV; van den Bergh Weerman, M. Invasion of lymphosarcoma cells into the perfused mouse liver. *J. Natl. Cancer Inst.*, 1977, 58, 399-407.
[116] Roos, E; Dingemans, KP; van de Pavert, IV; van den Bergh Weerman, MA. Mammary-carcinoma cells in mouse liver: infiltration of liver tissue and interaction with Kupffer cells. *Br. J. Cancer*, 1978, 38, 88-99.
[117] Dingemans, KP; Roos, E. Ultrastructural aspects of the invasion of liver by cancer cells (II). In: Weiss L, Gilbert HA, editors. *Liver metastasis*. Boston: G K Hall Medical Publishers; 1982; 51-76.
[118] Wallace, AC; Chew, EC; Jones, DS. Arrest and extravasation of cancer cells in the lung. In: Weiss L, Gilbert HA, editors. *Pulmonary metastasis*. Boston: G K Hall Medical Publishers; 1978; 26-42.

[119] Kinjo, M. Lodgement and extravasation of tumor cells in blood-borne metastasis: an electron microscope study. *Br. J. Cancer*, 1978, 38, 293-301.
[120] Chew, EC; Josephson, RL; Wallace, AC. Morphological aspects of the arrest of circulating cancer cells. In: Weiss L, editor. *Fundamental aspects of metastasis*. Amsterdam: North Holland; 1976; 121-150.
[121] Ludatscher, RM; Luse, SA; Suntzeff, V. An electron microscopic study of pulmonary tumor emboli from transplantable Morris hepatoma 5123. *Cancer Res.*, 1967, 27, 1939-1952.
[122] Warren, BA. Environment of the blood-borne tumor embolus adherent to vessel wall. *J. Med.*, 1973, 4, 150-177.

[123] Dingemans, KP; Roos, E; van den Bergh Weerman MA, van de Pavert IV. Invasion of liver tissue by tumor cells and leukocytes: comparative ultrastructure. *J. Natl. Cancer Inst.*, 1978, 60, 583-598.
[124] Marchesi, VT; Florey, HW. Electron micrographic observations on the emigration of leucocytes. *Q. J. Exp. Physiol. Coqn. Med. Sci.*, 1960, 45, 343-348.
[125] Machade, EA; Gerard, DA; Mitchell, JR; Lozzio, BB; Lozzio, CB. Arrest and extravasation of neoplastic cells: An electron microscopy study of serial sections at sequential stages. *Virchows Arch. Pathol. Anat.*, 1982, 396, 73-89.
[126] Azzarelli, B; Muller, J; Mirkin, LD; Goheen, MP. Transvascular migration of L2C leukemic cells studied in the liver of the guinea pig. *Virchows Arch. Pathol. Anat.*, 1985, 406, 425-440.
[127] Hori, K; Suzuki, M. Metastasis and blood vessel formation. *Mebio*, 1992, 9, 50-56. (in Japanese).
[128] Havrylov, S; Rzhepetskyy, Y; Malinowska, A; Drobot, L; Redowicz, MJ. Proteins recruited by SH3 domains of Ruk/CIN85 adaptor identified by LC-MS/MS. *Proteome Sci.*, 2009, 7, 1-19.
[129] Dvorak, AM; Feng, D. The vesiculo-vacuolar organelle (VVO): a new endothelial cell permeability organelle. *J. Histochem. Cytochem.*, 2001, 49, 419-432.
[130] Albiges-Rizo, C; Destaing, O; Fourcade, B; Planus, E; Block, MR. Actin machinery and mechanosensitivity in invadopodia, podosomes and focal adhesions. *J. Cell Sci.*, 2009, 122, 3037-3049.
[131] Poincloux, R; Lizárraga, F; Chavrier, P. Matrix invasion by tumour cells: a focus on MT1-MMP trafficking to invadopodia. *J. Cell Sci.*, 2009, 122, 3015-3024.
[132] Kawaguchi, T; Tobai, S; Nakamura, K. Cell surface structure of Yoshida sarcoma cells arrested in the liver sinusoids. In: Proceedings of the 39th annual meeting of the Japanese Cancer Association, Tokyo, 1980, 172.
[133] Witz, IP. The selectin-selectin ligand axis in tumor progression. *Cancer Metastasis Rev.*, 2008, 27, 19-30.
[134] Konno, A; Hoshino, Y; Terashima, S; Motoki, R; Kawaguchi, T. Carbohydrate expression profile of colorectal cancer cells is relevant to metastatic pattern and prognosis. *Clin. Exp. Metastasis*, 2002, 19, 61-70.
[135] Rosell, A; Cuadrado, E; Ortega-Aznar, A; Hernández-Guillamon, M; Lo, EH; Montaner, J. MMP-9-positive neutrophil infiltration is associated to blood-brain barrier breakdown and basal lamina type IV collagen degradation during hemorrhagic transformation after human ischemic

stroke. *Stroke*, 2008, 39, 1121-1126.

[136] Asahina, S. An experimental study on relationship between tumors and organs by direct transplantation of small number of cells of ascites tumors into tissues. *Fukushima Igaku Zashi*, 1967, 17, 65-89. (in Japanese).

[137] Dvorak, HF. Tumors: wounds that do not heal. Similarities between tumor stroma generation and wound healing. *N. Engl. J. Med.*, 1986, 315, 1650-1659.

[138] Krafts, KP. Tissue repair: The hidden drama. *Organogenesis*, 2010, 6, 225-233.

[139] Retsky, M. New concepts in breast cancer emerge from analyzing clinical data using numerical algorithms. *Int. J. Environ. Res. Public Health*, 2009, 6, 329-348.

[140] Fisher, B; Fisher, ER. Experimental evidence in support of the dormant tumor cells. *Science*, 1959, 130, 918-919.

[141] Luzzi, KJ; MacDonald, IC; Schmidt, EE; Kerkvliet, N; Morris, VL; Chambers, AF; Groom, AC. Multistep nature of metastatic inefficiency: dormancy of solitary cells after successful extravasation and limited survival of early micrometastases. *Am. J. Pathol.*, 1998, 153, 865-873.

[142] Folkman, J. The role of angiogenesis in tumor growth. *Semin. Cancer Biol.*, 1992, 3, 65-71.

[143] Goldfarb, Y; Ben-Eliyahu, S. Surgery as a risk factor for breast cancer recurrence and metastasis: mediating mechanisms and clinical prophylactic approaches. *Breast Dis.*, 2006-2007, 26, 99-114.

SECTION 2

ORGAN PREFERENCE METASTASIS

SUMMARY AND CONCLUSION

Tumor metastasis has two essential characteristics: "organ preference" and "differential metastatic potential." Organ preference metastasis means that every malignant tumor has unique organ distribution patterns of metastasis. We recently analyzed the correlations among these organ metastases by Pearson's correlation coefficient, which clearly showed that great difference exists among cancers with regard to organs affected by metastasis. In addition, we analyzed the metastatic distribution of pulmonary and gastric cancers. These results also demonstrated clear differences in metastatic organs by histological subtypes of these cancers. Two major hypothesis have been proposed based on the mechanisms involved in the organ preference in metastasis: the "seed-soil theory" and the "anatomical-mechanical theory." The seed and soil theory claims that metastasis occurs when tumor cell locates fertile tissue for easy growth. This hypothesis was opposed by the anatomical-mechanical hypothesis, which originally claimed that metastasis can be explained by the presence or absence of an anatomical connection that binds primary tumor and metastatic organ.

We have examined the distribution of metastatic foci of various kinds of animal tumor cells including B16 melanoma. From these results, we consider that the anatomical-mechanical hypothesis provides a reasonable explanation for preference in organ metastasis. However, anatomical-mechanical hypothesis could be explained at least in part by the microinjury hypothesis, proposing that circulating tumor cells preferentially produce metastases in injured tissues that were produced by tumor cell embolization. Tissue injury caused by tumor cell embolism may not only be limited to blood vessels, but also involves other tissues. This possibility was demonstrated by the facts that tumor metastasis was induced by embolization of dead tumor cells, ligation of blood vessels, or trauma. We suspect that tissue injury followed by the formation of granulation tissue provides a fertile soil for metastasis. We have performed a series of experimental studies using Yoshida sarcoma and a panel of rat ascites hepatoma induced by aminoazo dyes, in addition to B16 melanoma variant sublines. We selected sublines of eye, ovary, and bone from AH7974 cells, and the augmented metastatic potential of these sublines is linked each other, probably in relation to steroid hormone receptor expression. From the studies on the B16-14b and B16-B15b, we revealed that the preferential growth of these cells is related to their covering by meningothelial cells. Thus, we propose that the seed-soil hypothesis and the anatomical-mechanical hypothesis are not conflicting ones, but these hypothesis explain what kinds of “soil” tumor cell prefer.

We need further information on organ preference metastasis in order to extend our knowledge on clinical cases in accordance to TNM classification, origin and differentiation of tumor cells, and tissue district of target organs.

INTRODUCTION

Tumor metastasis is the most important characteristic of malignant tumors. For a considerable time, many researchers have tried to elucidate the determinant(s) involved in metastasis, but metastasis is an extremely complex phenomenon, and to date, they have not been able to identify a definite determinant for all malignant tumors [1, 2]. We believe that tumor metastasis has two essential characteristics: “organ preference” and “differential metastatic potential” [3, 4], and these characteristics require detailed clarification to elucidate the determinant(s) in metastasis.

Chapter III

Demonstration of Organ Preference in Metastasis Through Analysis of Human Cancers in Autopsy Cases

Table 6 shows the representative organ or tissue distribution of metastatic tumors in autopsy cases as determined in our laboratory. This distribution pattern is basically identical to data collected by researchers in other laboratories over different periods. Based on these data, it is apparent that different tumors show similarity with regard to organs targeted by metastasis. For example, lung, liver, adrenal gland, bone, and lymph nodes are frequently involved in metastasis.

We recently analyzed the correlations among these organ metastases by Pearson's correlation coefficient, which clearly showed that great differences exist among tumors with regard to organs affected by metastasis (Figure 39) [5].

In addition, we analyzed the metastatic distribution of lung cancer and gastric cancer to the lung, liver, bone, and adrenal gland from the standpoint of histological subtypes. These results also demonstrated clear differences in metastatic organs by histological subtypes of lung cancer and gastric cancer (Figure 40) [6]. Therefore, we believe that all malignant tumors metastasize to similar organs/tissues, but each of them has a unique metastatic propensity.

Two major hypothesis have been proposed based on the mechanisms involved in the organ preference in metastasis: the "seed–soil theory" and the "anatomical–mechanical theory." In 1889, Paget [7] proposed and explained the seed–soil theory mechanism. This hypothesis claims that metastasis occurs when tumor cells locate fertile tissue for easy growth.

Table 6. Distribution of metastasis of major types of malignant tumors autopsied at Fukushima Medical University School of Medicine

Organ or tissue	Leukemia (170 cases)	Multiple myeloma (44 cases)	Malignant lymphoma (77 cases)	Lung cancer (143 cases)	Esophageal cancer (41 cases)	Gastric cancer (154 cases)	Carcinoma of large intestine (71 cases)	Hepatocellular carcinoma (61 cases)	Carcinoma of bile duct (40 cases)
Brain	6.5	-	4.0	13.3	2.4	-	4.2	1.7	-
Hypophysis	1.8	-	-	0.7	-	-	-	-	-
Meninges	7.6	-	5.3	-	-	-	-	-	-
Leptomeninges	-	-	-	2.8	-	3.2	-	-	-
Dura mater	-	-	-	1.4	-	1.3	1.4	-	-
Thyroid gland	4.2	2.3	5.3	8.4	7.3	1.9	2.8	-	2.5
Thymus	3.6	-	5.3	-	-	-	-	-	-
Tongue	3.0	2.3	8.0	-	-	-	-	-	-
Tonsil	14.4	4.5	17.3	-	-	-	-	-	-
Heart	18.0	-	8.0	5.6	2.4	1.3	1.4	-	-
Pericardium (carcinom atous pericarditis)	6	-	24	14.7	4.9	6.5	1.4	-	-
Lung (opposite lung)	40.1	20.5	49.3	(50.3)	39.0	40.9	45.1	50.9	35.0
Pleura (carcinomatous pleuritis)	2.4	6.8	14.7	20.3	14.6	16.2	8.5 (5.6)	3.5	15
Liver	54.5	38.6	61.3	49.0	22.0	41.6	49.3	40.0	42.5
Gallbladder	-	-	-	-	-	-	-	-	-
Paritoneum (carcinom atous peritonitis)	1.2	-	10.7	4.9	7.3	34.4 (16.2)	26.8 (21.1)	19.3	25.0
Diaphragm	-	-	-	-	-	-	-	-	-
Spleen	71.3	54.5	53.3	6.3	-	5.8	2.8	1.7	5.0
Pancreas	11.4	4.5	25.3	11.2	4.9	9.7	4.2	-	-
Kidney	43.1	15.9	56.7	22.4	7.3	10.4	4.2	1.7	10.0
Adrenal gland	16.2	15.9	29.3	42.0	7.3	24.7	25.4	10.5	22.5
Esophagus	7.3	-	4.0	0.7	12.2	-	-	-	-
Stomach	13.3	4.5	26.7	4.2	-	-	-	-	-
Intestine	21.3	11.4	36.0	7.7	-	-	-	-	-
Urinary bladder	6.6	-	8.0	2.1	-	-	-	-	-
Prostate	4.8	-	14.6	0.7	-	-	-	-	-
Testis	17.9	9.1	19.2	-	-	-	-	-	-
Ovary	21.8	4.5	12.5	2.1	-	30.6	3.6	-	4.2
Uterus	14.3	-	-	1.4	-	10.2	3.6	-	-
Vagina	-	-	-	-	-	-	-	-	-
Bone/bone marrow	84.2	90.5	50.0	41.3	7.3	24.0	16.9	15.8	12.5
Lymph node	46.7	34.1	75.3	76.2	51.2	66.2	36.6	24.6	65.0
Skeletal muscle/muscle	1.8	4.5	-	0.7	-	-	-	-	-
Skin	6.6	4.5	8.0	6.3	2.4	6.5	2.8	-	-

Organ or tissue	Pancreatic cancer (40 cases)	Renal cell carcinoma (27 cases)	Prostatic cancer # (28 cases)	Uterine cervical cancer (106 cases)	Ovarian cancer (30 cases)	Choriocarcinoma (22 cases)	Thyroid cancer (46 cases)	Breast cancer (97 cases)
Brain	-	22.2	7.1(12.5)	1.9	3.3	72.7	2.1	15.5
Hypophysis	-	3.7	3.6(6.3)	1.0	-	-	-	6.2
Meninges	-	-	-	-	3.3	-	-	-
Leptomeninges	-	-	-	-	-	-	-	3.1
Dura mater	-	-	-	3.8	-	-	4.3	12.4
Thyroid gland	-	7.4	-	2.8	3.3	4.5	-	14.4
Thymus	-	-	-	-	-	-	-	-
Tongue	-	-	-	-	-	-	-	-
Tonsil	-	-	-	-	-	-	-	-
Heart	8.1	11.1	-	3.8	-	-	2.1	4.1
Pericardium (carcinom atous pericarditis)	2.7	3.7	-	3.8	6.7	4.5	4.3	13.4
Lung (opposite lung)	48.6	48.1	39.6(68.8)	40.6	26.7	100.0	47.8	80.4
Pleura (carcinomatous pleuritis)	18.9(16.2)	18.5	12.9(25.0)	6.6	26.7	4.5	10.9	39.2
Liver	62.2	18.5	25.0(43.8)	27.4	46.7	31.8	15.2	70.1
Gallbladder	-	-	-	-	-	-	-	-
Paritoneum (carcinom atous peritonitis)	43.2(5.4)	3.7	-	23.6	66.7	-	4.3	7.2
Diaphragm	-	-	-	4.7	-	4.5	-	-
Spleen	8.1	-	-	2.8	13.3	18.2	-	12.4
Pancreas	-	7.4	7.1(12.5)	4.7	-	9.1	4.3	12.4
Kidney	13.5	11.1	17.4(31.3)	12.3	3.3	59.1	8.7	16.5
Adrenal gland	29.7	25.9	17.9(31.3)	9.4	20.0	4.5	8.7	46.4
Esophagus	-	-	-	-	-	-	2.1	-
Stomach	-	-	-	1.9	-	4.5	-	-
Intestine	-	-	-	2.8	-	40.9	2.1	6.2
Urinary bladder	-	-	-	1.9	-	-	-	1.0
Prostate	-	-	※	※	※	-	-	-
Testis	-	-	-	※	※	※	-	※
Ovary	2.7	-	※	4.7	-	-	-	13.4
Uterus	-	-	※	-	3.3	-	-	11.3
Vagina	-	-	※	-	3.3	-	-	-
Bone/bone marrow	32.4	37.0	42.9(75.0)	18.9	6.7	18.2	15.2	67.0
Lymph node	78.3	44.4	46.4(81.3)	56.6	50.0	27.3	41.3	76.3
Skeletal muscle/muscle	-	7.4	-	-	-	4.5	-	-
Skin	-	14.8	-	2.8	16.7	4.5	6.5	34.0

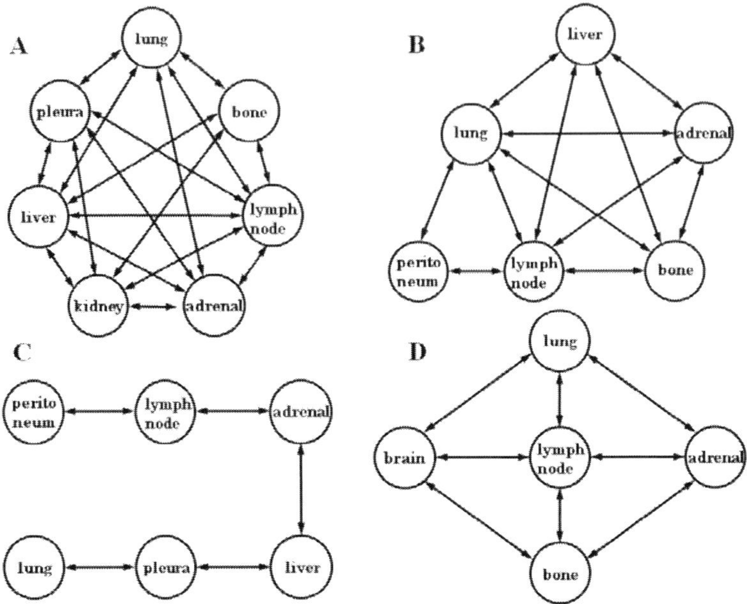

Figure 39. Correlation of organ metastasis in human cancer. Pearson's correlation coefficient was obtained in all cases involving two organs with frequency of metastasis >20%. Lines connect organs with significant relationship ($p < 0.05$). A, B, C, and D show data for lung, stomach, ovary, and renal cell cancers, respectively [4].

The seed–soil hypothesis is supported by several researchers who mainly studied malignant melanoma cells, including human specimens [1, 2, 8]. This hypothesis was opposed by the anatomical–mechanical hypothesis, which claimed that organ preference in metastasis can be explained by the presence or absence of an anatomical connection that binds primary tumor and metastatic organ and/or physiological properties of tumor cells, such as size/cluster. This hypothesis was proposed before the seed-soil hypothesis and was supported by Ewing in 1928 [9], followed by Walther [10] in 1948, who proposed a scheme by which metastatic distribution is explained. In recent years, this hypothesis has been overtaken by the cascade theory, which was proposed by Viadana [11] in 1978. In conjunction with the paravertebral venous system proposed by Batson [12], this hypothesis seems to be widely accepted at present.

Through our studies and others based on analysis of human autopsy cases, we believe that some cases of metastasis can be explained by the seed–soil hypothesis, but others could equally be explained by the anatomical–mechanical hypothesis.

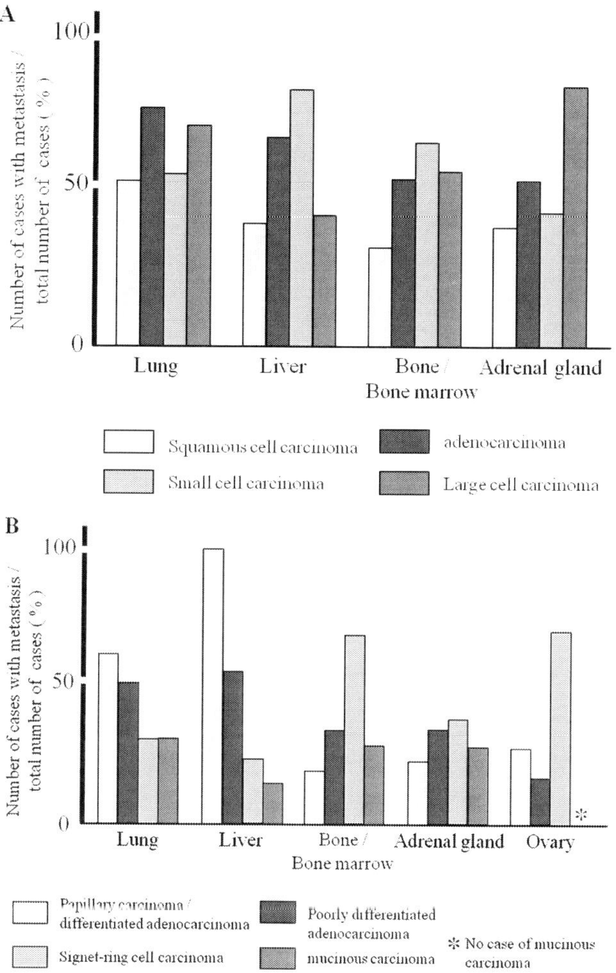

Figure 40. A: Metastatic distribution of lung cancer according to histological subtype. B: Metastatic distribution of gastric cancer according to histological subtype. There are marked differences in organ preference in metastasis among histological subtypes [Kawaguchi T., unpublished data].

The key to the argument surrounding the two hypothesis is the issue of metastatic tumor growth: the seed–soil hypothesis claims the micro-environment-dependent nature of metastatic tumor growth, while the anatomical–mechanical hypothesis argues for autonomous growth ability of metastatic tumor cells. Therefore, we performed experimental studies on organ preference in metastasis, as described below.

Chapter IV

EXPERIMENTAL VERIFICATION OF ORGAN PREFERENCE IN METASTASIS

Considering all sources of human, extensive experimental models have been developed, and studies have been performed to clarify the existence of organ preference metastasis and the mechanisms involved in it.

1. ANATOMICAL-MECHANICAL AND MICROINJURY HYPOTHESIS

1.1. Anatomical-Mechanical Hypothesis

One of the facts supporting the anatomical–mechanical hypothesis on distribution of organ preference in metastasis is that metastasis frequently occurs in organs/tissues connected by blood vessels through which tumor cells are injected. Fundamentally, this situation is the same in both lymphatic and celomic metastases. For example, metastatic tumor colonies were formed in the lung when tumor cells were injected via the tail vein. On the other hand, metastases occurred in the liver when tumor cells were injected via the portal vein. Injection of tumor cells into the left ventricle of the heart yielded tumor colonies in various organs/tissues, including the brain. Table 7 shows our own experimental results on organ colonization distribution by a subline of B16B-15b [13]. This subline formed tumor nodules in the thoracic cavity, including the lungs, as well as in the brain meninges when tumor cells were injected via the tail vein. When rat ascites cell line AH130 was injected into the liver, tumor cells metastasized not only to the omentum and peritoneum but also to the lung. Interestingly, the AH130 cell line has also been shown to metastasize to the adrenal glands, which are the preferred site of metastasis in this tumor line [14]. Therefore, we consider that the anatomical–mechanical hypothesis provides a reasonable explanation, at least in part, for preference in organ metastasis.

Table 7. Distribution pattern of tumors after injection of B16-B15b cells via the tail vein, left ventricle of the heart, or left carotid artery

	Number of animals with tumors/total number of animals [a]		
	B16:B15b		
Tumor site	i.v. [b]	i.c. [c]	i.a. [d]
Brain			
Meninges	5/8 [e]	7/7	8/8
Ventricle	0/8	3/7	5/8
Choroid plexus	0/8	1/7	0/8
Parenchyma	0/8	1/7	7/8
Heart	0/8	6/7	0/8
Thoracic cavity	8/8	6/7	1/8
Liver	0/8	0/7	0/8
Spleen	0/8	4/7	0/8
Pancreas	0/8	1/7	0/8
Kidney	3/8 [e]	2/7	0/8
Adrenal gland	1/8	7/7	0/8
Ovary	3/8	6/7	0/8
Uterus	0/8	0/7	0/8
Lymph nodes	0/8	2/7	0/8
Subcutaneous	0/8	1/7	1/8
Cervical (submandibular)	0/8	0/7	4/8
Other sites	0/8	0/7	2/8 [f]
Lung	8/8	7/7	8/8
Av. No. lung tumor colonies (range)	92(32–160)	11(0–62)	5(0–20)
Av. day autopsy (range) [g]	27(25–28) [h]	22(19–27)	20(17–27)

[a]: 0.1 ml of a single tumor cell suspension containing 5×10^4 cells was injected into each female C57BL6 mouse. [b]: Tail vein. [c]: Left ventricle of the heart. [d]: Left common carotid artery. [e]: Tumor growth was found mainly in the blood vessels with invasion into perivascular tissue. [f]: 2/8 orbital. [g]: All animals were sacrificed 28 days post-injection. [h]: Three animals died with tumors from 25 to 27 days post-injection, and the remaining five animals were sacrificed at 28 days post-injection [13].

In addition, other experimental examples support the anatomical–mechanical hypothesis. For example, spheroidal C3H mouse mammary carcinoma cells formed more metastatic lung tumors than that with a single tumor cell suspension [15], and AH100B rat ascites tumor cells did not form metastatic tumors in post-pulmonary organs/tissues when tumor cells were injected via the tail vein [16].

Tumor cell cluster resistance against a leukocyte attack in the metastatic tumor growth was suggested as the mechanism in the former example. Reduced likelihood of less deformable AH109A passing through pulmonary capillary beds was suggested as the mechanism in the latter example.

1.2. Limitations of the Anatomical-Mechanical Hypothesis and Proposal of Microinjury Hypothesis

It is necessary to scrutinize the relationship between the passage of tumor cells through organ capillary beds and metastasis formation, since Zeidman demonstrated that tumor cells can pass through capillary beds [17], and Coman et al. claimed that the metastatic site does not necessarily correspond to tumor cell embolization [18]. Thus, we believe that there is a need to determine certain anatomical–mechanical factors, which will help the tumor cells to form metastases.

We consider that the anatomical–mechanical hypothesis could be explained, at least in part, by the microinjury hypothesis, with regard to three bodies of experimental work. The first of these was carried out by Suzuki [19], who found that the occurrence of brain metastasis by the injection of rat ascites hepatoma cells was dependent to a large extent on the presence of islands (tumor cell clusters) in hepatoma cell lines. This is because brain (parenchyma) metastasis did not occur with the free-cell type of tumor line but did with island-formed cell types.

Following on Suzuki's experiment, Asahina [20] injected a small number of rat ascites hepatoma cells (10, 100, and 1000 cells) into the brain and investigated the correlation between tumor take in the brain and brain parenchyma metastasis formation. However, he failed to demonstrate any correlation between them.

We examined the transcerebral passage of tumor cells and its relationship to brain parenchyma metastasis using Yoshida sarcoma and six strains of rat ascites hepatoma (Figure 41 and [21]). These tumors could be subdivided into "island (i.e., cell cluster)-forming strains" (AH130, AH272, and AH7974) and “single-cell strains” (Yoshida sarcoma, AH7974F, and AH13). We found that the island-forming strains showed a low passage rate through the cerebral capillaries and readily produced metastases, while the single-cell strains showed a high passage rate and rarely formed metastases. Thus, we discovered that the incidence of arrested tumor cells corresponded directly to the frequency of developing tumors (Figure 41).

From these studies, we suggest that any microinjury foci could be produced by the larger emboli of the island-forming strains. Rapid passage of tumor cells through the brain would result in minimal injury (Figure 41).

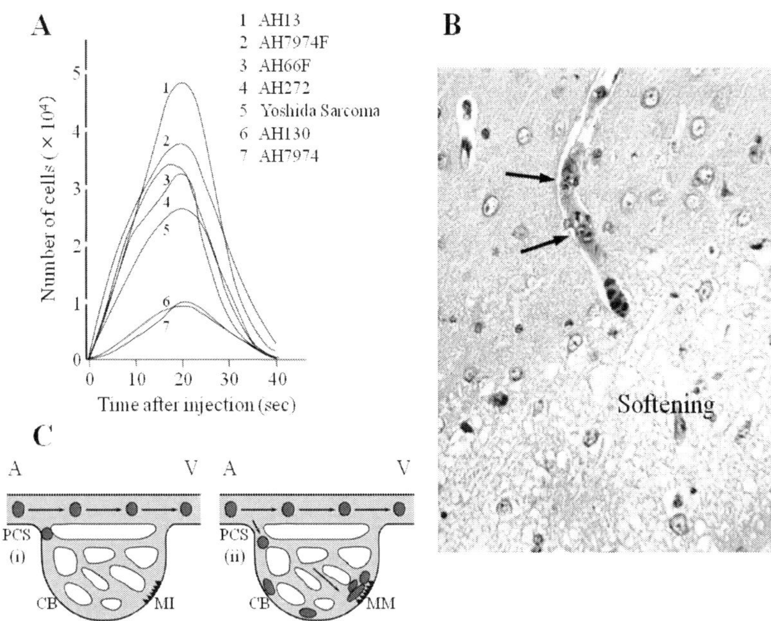

Figure 41. Brain metastasis and microinjury hypothesis. A: Transcerebral passage of rat ascites hepatoma cells. Brain parenchymal metastasis occurred with AH130 and AH7974 showing lower transcerebral passage rates, whereas brain metastasis rarely occurred with strains showing higher transcerebral passage rates [21]. B: Tumor cells (AH7974) embolized in a cerebral capillary at arrows and induced softening of cerebral tissue. C: The microinjury hypothesis: a tumor cell with lower transcerebral passage rate in an arteriole (A) embolized in the precapillary sphincter (PCS). The embolism resulted in the spasm of the blood vessel, which followed microinjury (MI) of the dominant capillary bed (CB). Tumor cells lodged in the damaged CB and formed a micrometastasis (MM). In contrast, tumor cells with higher transcerebral passage rates rarely formed MI in capillary beds because of their weak embolization properties [cited from reference 22]. (V): venule.

Warren [22] contributed the following information to our results: (1) tumor cells can pass through intact circulation beds without arrest and without producing metastasis; (2) the development of tumor is dose-dependent: below a certain number of tumor cells, metastasis will not occur, and this number varies for each individual tumor; and (3) circulating tumor cells preferentially produce metastases in injured tissues. He named it "the microinjury hypothesis," and we used the term in this book.

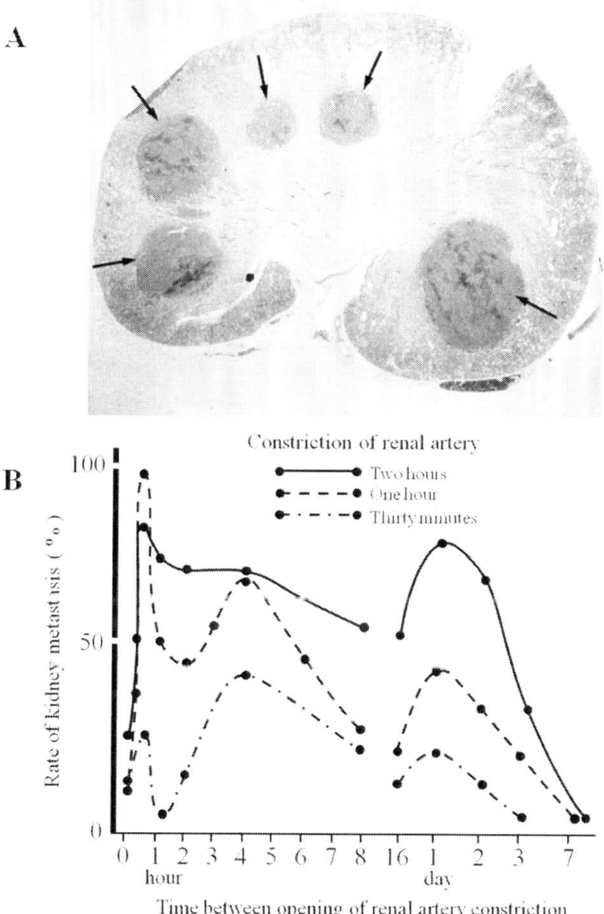

Figure 42. Induction of metastasis in the kidney by ischemia. A: Macroscopic appearance of induced metastasis. Five metastatic nodules were seen in the medulla of the kidney, 14 days after injection of rat ascites hepatoma AH130 cells (arrow). B: Effects of ischemia on renal artery constriction and reflow following metastasis [23].

1.3. From Microinjury Hypothesis to Tissue Injury Hypothesis with Regard to Organ Preference in Metastasis

Tissue injury caused by tumor cell embolism may not only be limited to blood vessels but also involves other tissues. This possibility was demonstrated by the following studies on histological and electron microscopic analyses of injured tissues and induction of tumor metastasis by embolization of dead tumor cells, ligation of blood vessels, or trauma (Figure 42) [23–26]. From these studies, along with others [27–29], we propose three phases in the microinjury hypothesis in relation to metastasis formation. Phase 1 is associated with the lodgment of tumor cells in injured blood vessels, especially blood capillaries and post-capillary venules. This phase may require a few minutes to an hour after tumor embolization. The affected blood vessels include capillaries and/or post-capillary venules, while fibrin deposition and leukocyte adhesion occurred in these vessels. Phase 2 is associated with the extravasation of tumor cells lodged in injured blood vessels. The time after embolization is considerably variable, depending on the tissues/organs involved, and it ranges from about 4 to 72 hours. This variation was likely to be caused by the properties of tissues and the construction of affected blood vessels. This phase may be correlated with blood vessel permeability. Phase 3 involved the repair of injured tissues with various types of cell and the association of immature granulation tissue and tumor growth. This final phase varies considerably in time frame, sometimes continuing for up to three weeks. We suspect that tissue injury followed by the formation of granulation tissue provides a fertile base for extravasated tumor cell growth, through both abundant vascular networks and the release of several kinds of growth factor related to tissue regeneration [30]. Growth factors in tissue injury and granulation tissues include EGF, TGF, HGF (SF), FGF, PDGF, and IGF.

Thus, considering that injury to tissues affected by tumor cell embolism is not limited to vascular walls, the microinjury hypothesis should be termed as “the tissue injury hypothesis”; in fact, recent experimental studies support our hypothesis. For example, Orr et al. [31] and Soares et al. [32] reported that neutrophil- and/or free radical-mediated microvascular injury can promote organ localization and metastasis by circulating tumor cells. At present, we are unsure whether the microinjury/tissue injury hypothesis can explain organ preference in metastasis in human cancers. However, it is likely that the lung and liver are frequently affected by tumor cell embolisms resulting in an injured tissue predisposing to metastasis formation. Metastases in the brain and adrenal glands are frequently formed in the junctional areas of the cortex and medulla, supporting the microinjury hypothesis of organ preference metastasis. In recent years, some clinicians have claimed that clinical trials of interleukin 1 (IL-1) blockade should be initiated for cancer patients to investigate the prevention of metastasis [33].

2. SEED-SOIL HYPOTHESIS

Appropriate experimental systems are necessary to verify the seed-soil hypothesis. To date, three types of cell lines have been used to study the seed-soil hypothesis: 1) transplantable tumor cell line, 2) in vivo/in vitro-selected sublines from a transplantable tumor cell line, and 3) gene-transfected tumor cell lines. The first cell line type demonstrates organ preference metastasis: in this category, we identified 40 mouse tumor cell lines, ten rat tumor cell lines, and several cell lines from guinea pigs, rabbits, and humans, almost ten years before [34]. Almost all of these cell lines are spontaneously derived during serial transplantation of original cells or following carcinogen administration. The second cell line type is selected in vivo-in vivo or in vivo-in vitro from the first cell line type. We identified around 20 lines established from the in vivo–in vivo selection procedure and around ten lines from in vivo–in vitro selection procedure [35]. The third type example is found in the study of Matsuura et al. [36], who transfected integrin α4 cDNA to CHO cells for developing bone metastasis sublines.

We performed a series of experimental studies using Yoshida sarcoma and a panel of rat ascites hepatoma induced by aminoazo dyes [37]. The origin of Yoshida sarcoma remained uncertain for a long time, but it is now considered to be an ascites hepatoma [38]. Around 60 distinct lines of rat ascites hepatoma are maintained in Japanese laboratories and have been utilized in various types of cancer research, including metastasis [39]. Every cell line exhibits not only a particular cellular phenotype but also characteristic metastatic distribution.

2.1. Rat Ascites Hepatoma AH7974 and Its Variant Subline AH7974F

Rat ascites hepatoma AH7974 is an "island-forming cell line" that produces few cell aggregate-like islands in a single cell. This cell line metastasizes to the parenchyma, ventricle, and choroid plexus of the brain, the lung, and the adrenal gland when injected into the carotid artery, tail vein, or left ventricle, but they rarely metastasize to the liver, even when injected into the portal vein. On the contrary, AH7974F cells, a subline of AH7974, were discovered during the process of serial intraperitoneal (ip) transplantation. This cell line generally metastasizes to the liver but rarely to the brain, irrespective of the route of injection (Tables 2, 3; Figures 23-25, 41) [40]. When tumor cells were injected into the carotid artery, the number of AH7974 cells detected in the brain was approximately ten times more than that of AH7974F cells.

Conversely, the number of AH7974 cells detected in the liver was ~10 times less than that of AH7974F cells. The arrest of these cells in the brain vasculature is associated with microinjury of the vasculature, as described above, while the arrest of these cells in the liver is mainly caused by direct adhesion to the endothelial cells and/or Kupffer cells.

Two interesting events occur in the growth of AH7974 and AH7974F cells during these metastatic processes. First, there is an exponential growth of AH7974 in the brain parenchyma due to decreased cell loss after extravasation of tumor cells. On the other hand, the AH7974F cells lodged in the brain vasculature, which are incapable of extravasation, die. In the liver, in contrast, the AH7974F cells extravasate from the sinusoidal vessels and proliferate in the liver parenchyma without a loss in number, whereas the AH7974 cells are incapable of extravasation and die within the blood vasculature (Chapter I, Section 4).

The second event is the difference in the growth kinetics of the AH7974F cells in the brain and liver, which we examined through grain dilution of tritiated thymidine by the AH7974F cells. This clearly demonstrated the AH7974F cell division in the liver but not in the brain parenchyma. We also noticed a similar difference in the proliferation kinetics of the AH7974 cells: when injected into the carotid artery, the AH7974 cells formed only small metastatic nodules in the brain parenchyma but large ones in the choroid plexus of the ventricles; in the choroid plexus, these cells showed higher labeling indices of tritiated thymidine than in the brain parenchyma [41-43].

Sato [44] analyzed the differences between AH7974 and AH7974F cells by the genomic scanning method and found 14 more expression spots in AH7974F than in AH7974 when 1,200 spots were compared. One of these was considered to be tropomyosin, but the remainder was not identified. It should be noted here that this unfavorable nature of the metastatic soil of the liver for the AH7974 cells and the brain for the AH7974F cells easily becomes favorable by various types of tissue injury (Figure 43).

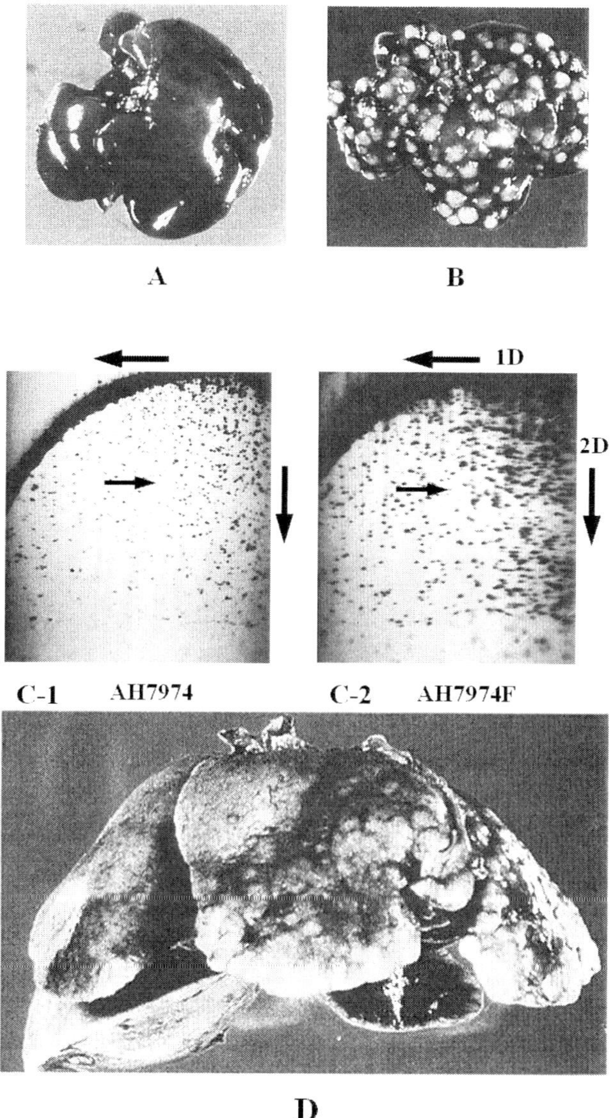

Figure 43. Rat ascites hepatoma AH7974F was derived from AH7974. AH7974 cells never metastasize to the liver, irrespective of route of inoculation, including the portal vein (A). On the other hand, AH7974F metastasize to the liver severely, irrespective of route of inoculation (B). When the difference was examined by the genomic scanning method, there were differences in 14 spots among approximately 1,200 examined (C). One of these was tropomyosin, and the remainder was not identified [44]. The metastatic propensities of AH7974 and AH7974F cells are easily lost through tissue injury [25], as AH7974 cells metastasized to injured liver tissue (D).

2.2. Brain Meninges Metastasis by B16 Melanoma Sublines

When a tumor is composed of heterogeneous mixed subpopulations, and organ preference metastasis property of the tumor cells is genetically stable, the subpopulation can be chosen. In 1973, Fidler [45] reported on the subline (B16-F1~F10) of B16 melanoma, highly metastatic for the lung, by in vivo–in vitro selection procedures. Since then, many variant sublines displaying high organ specificity and metastatic potential have been reported [46]. These selection studies have elucidated the organ preference metastasis and the molecules involved in the process [47]. However, there are several unanswered questions about the significance of metastasis formation, especially with regard to organ preference metastasis. Here, we describe our own studies concerning metastatic variant sublines that were selected from Fidler's original procedures [13, 48].

Nicolson et al. [49] selected and established several brain preference metastasis sublines from the B16 melanoma cells, including B16-B14b and B16-B15b, by the in vitro–in vivo selection procedure. Both B16-B14b and B16-B15b metastasize to the brain surface (meninges), lung, ovary, and adrenal gland (Table 7, Figure 44) [13]. Therefore, these sublines are not "brain-specific." There is both a similarity and a difference in the brain metastatic propensity between these cell lines. The high incidence of brain surface metastasis is similar in both the cell lines, but it is the size of the metastases that divides them: B16-B15b cells invariably form large tumor colonies, while those associated with B16-B14b are generally very small.

Since hematogenous brain metastasis is achieved by lodgment, extravasation, and growth, Nicolson et al. have further demonstrated that brain-selected metastatic cells selectively adhere to the brain-derived endothelial cells, migrate to the chemotactic factor derived from these endothelial cells, and express transferrin receptor [49]. We are interested in the different host cell responses in/around the metastatic foci of both cell lines; metastatic nodules associated with B16-B14b cells include many fibroblasts and lymphocytes, whereas such a host cell reaction is rare or infrequent in nodules associated with B16-B15b [48]. In addition, we observed that B16-B15b cell metastatic nodules were well-covered by meningothelial cells, but B16-B14b cell nodules were not. These histopathological findings suggest that brain surface metastatic tumor formation is strongly influenced by the lymphocytic response of these cell lines and an interaction between tumor cells and meningothelial cells. However, further studies on the role of host cell reactions in organ preference metastasis formation are required.

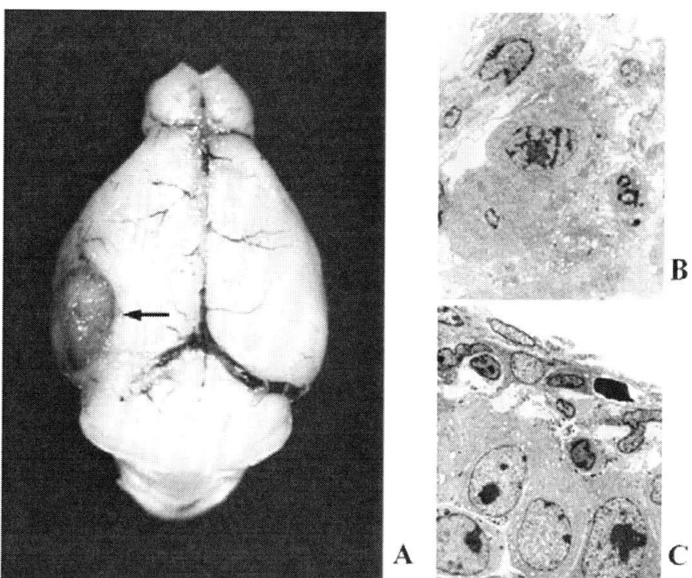

Figure 44. B16-B14b and B16-B15b. A: Gross appearance of brain meninges metastatic tumor of B16-B15b. The tumor was located in dura mater and did not invade into brain parenchyma. B: Electron microscopic examination revealed that B16-14b brain meninges tumor was accompanied by lymphocytic infiltration and remained small. C: On the other hand, meninges tumor of B16-B15b was big and usually covered by meningothelial cells on the surface. The lymphocytic infiltration of lymphocytic cells was a few [13, 48].

Nevertheless, we found that splenectomy or laparotomy following implantation of tumor cells enhanced the growth of brain meningeal tumor nodules [48], but more information will be needed before any generalization can be made.

2.3. Eye, Ovary, and Bone Metastasis Associated with Rat Ascites Hepatoma Sublines

Rat ascites hepatoma cell line AH7974 metastasizes to the eye, ovary, adrenal gland, and bone, but at low frequency. This metastatic propensity has been stable for about 30 years. We obtained metastatic sublines from the eye, ovary, and bone by Fidler's in vivo–in vitro (left ventricle (iv) injection) selection procedure and compared the metastatic propensity among them (Table 8 and Figure 45) [50-52].

A. Eye Metastasis Subline

When inoculated into the left cardiac ventricle, ten times-selected variant cells (74E10) formed metastasis in the rat eye at 90% frequency. In contrast, the incidence of eye metastasis for the parental line (74E0) was <10%. Cell line 74E10 also metastasized to the ovary and adrenal gland at high frequency compared to the parental 74E0, although the eye was the most preferred site. Metastatic tumors associated with 74E10 grew more aggressively than those of 74E0, although both had similar in vitro growth rate. Karyotype analysis revealed altered chromosome numbers: 74E0 showed diploid and 74E10 showed hypertriploid chromosomes (Figure 51). The level of neuraminidase-accessible sialic acid on the 74E10 tumor surface was twice of 74E10. However, there were no apparent differences in the incidences and distribution of metastases between neuraminidase-treated and untreated 74E10 cells. Thymectomy and splenectomy a week prior to intraventricular injection of 74E10 cells did not influence the incidence and distribution of metastases.

B. Ovary Metastasis Subline

When AH7974 cell line was injected by left ventricle route, ovarian metastasis was found in 3 of 29 rats (~11%). When in vivo–in vitro selection was repeated six times, all the examined rats exhibited ovarian metastasis (10/10). Incidence and size of ovarian tumor reached a maximum with six (OV6) and seven times-selected procedures (OV7), respectively (Table 8B and Figure 45).

During these experiments, the chromosome number of tumor cells changed from diploid (AH7974, OV1-OV5) to tetraploid (OV6-OV10) (Figure 51). OV7 cells lodged and proliferated preferentially in the newly formed corpus luteum in which the tumor cells were in close contact with lutein cells via their microvilli. It was observed that the tumor cells sometimes contained lipid-like droplets similar to those in lutein cells. The incidence of metastasis in OV7 cells in visceral organs other than the ovary showed no distinct difference among rats of ovariectomized and non-ovariectomized female and male groups.

Estrogen and progesterone had no effect on the proliferation of OV7 cells in vitro, but they inhibited cell proliferation under high concentrations. Estrogen receptor and progesterone receptor were not detected in any cell lines of AH7974, OV1, and OV7 by the radioreceptor assay. However, when the receptor was examined by the avidin–biotin complex (ABC) method, we found a progesterone receptor-positive sign in OV7 cells metastasized in the ovary (Figure 45D).

C. Bone Metastasis Subline

AH7974 cells rarely metastasize to the bones (vertebrae, femur, and scapula).

Table 8. Establishment of eye-, ovary- and bone-selected metastatic variant sublines of rat ascites hepatoma AH7974 and linkage of each cell line in organ preference metastasis

A. Eye metastatic variants											
Metastatic site	AH7974	E1	E2	E3	E4	E5	E6	E7	E8	E9	E10
Eye	7	10	33	70	40	80	42	80	60	60	90
Brain	14	0	17	40	0	20	0	50	50	0	23
Lung	0	0	0	0	0	0	0	40	30	0	20
Adrenal gland	39	10	58	10	20	50	17	60	70	60	70
Ovary	15	0	42	30	30	60	8	50	60	30	63
No. of animals examined	56	10	12	10	10	10	12	10	10	10	30
B. Ovary metastatic variants											
Metastatic site	AH7974	OV1	OV2	OV3	OV4	OV5	OV6	OV7	OV8	OV9	OV10
Ovary	3	11	60	80	40	80	100	100	90	90	80
Brain	7	11	60	70	60	80	50	80	70	60	52
Lung	0	38	70	80	30	80	30	10	100	100	58
Adrenal gland	20	44	70	90	50	80	80	100	90	90	88
Eye	0	0	70	90	20	80	40	100	70	90	76
Kidney	0	0	40	50	30	30	40	80	44	70	28
Liver	0	0	0	0	0	0	0	0	0	0	0
spleen	0	0	0	0	0	0	0	0	0	0	0
No. of animals examined	29	9	10	10	10	10	10	10	10	10	25

C. Bone metastatic variants					
Metastatic site	AH7974	Bo-1	Bo-2	Bo-3	Bo-4
Bone					
Sternum	0	33	10	90	100
Rib	0	50	30	30	100
Vertebral bone	13	83	20	100	100
Femur	13	67	60	100	100
Scapular bone	13	17	10	0	20
Ovary	63	67	60	100	100
Adrenal gland	63	50	70	100	100
Lung	38	50	40	100	90
Brain	38	0	30	70	100
Eye	25	0	0	90	80
Kidney	25	17	0	0	0
Pancreas	0	17	10	0	0
Liver	0	0	0	0	0
Spleen	0	0	0	0	0
Lymph nodes	25	83	60	90	90

Cell lines metastasizing to the bone were cultured in vitro and injected into the left ventricle of rats. When the procedure was repeated four times, the cell line (Bo-4) was highly metastatic to the bone, as well as to the lung, ovary, adrenal gland, brain, and lymph node (Table 8 and Figure 45). Detailed histological examinations revealed that metastasis had initially occurred in the bone marrow of the epiphysis. Chromosome number and doubling time of Bo-4 cell growth were similar to those of the parent AH7974 (Figure 51). Immunohistochemical evaluation of cell blocks from cultures and blocks of metastatic foci from the bone and lung showed decreased expression of fibronectin receptor and progesterone receptor, and no changes in expression were detected with regard to fibronectin cell-binding protein, laminin receptor, vitronectin receptor, E-cadherin, estrogen receptor, and p53 protein.

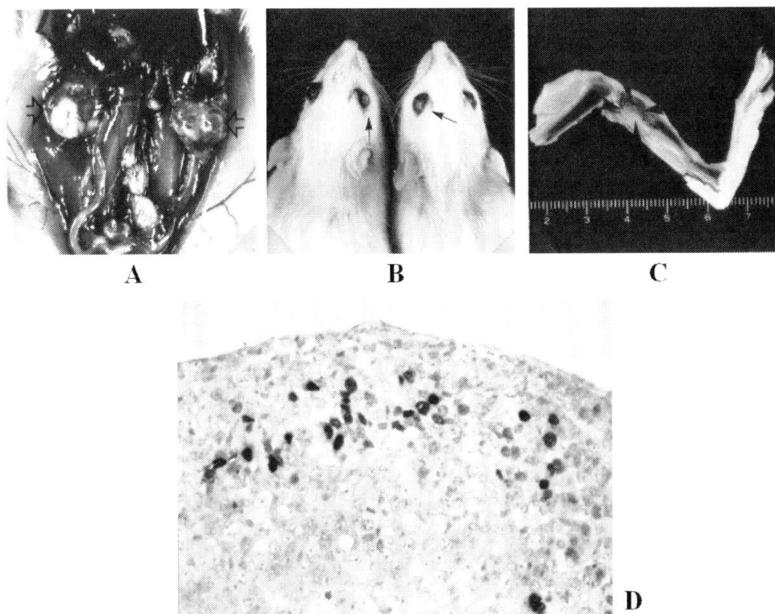

Figure 45. Organ preference metastasis of rat ascites hepatoma cell line AH7974 and its variant sublines. Rat ascites hepatoma AH7974 cells rarely metastasize to the eye, ovary, and bone, irrespective of the route of transplantation. When metastatic tumor cells from the ovary (A), eye (B), and bone (C) were cultured in vitro and injected, large tumors formed in the respective organs. Cells selected from any of these three organs frequently formed large tumors in the other two. These three lines appear to have common mechanisms of organ preference metastasis. D: Ovarian metastatic foci containing estrogen receptor-positive tumor cells [50-52].

From the above results, we conclude that the rat ascites hepatoma AH7974 cell line shows organ preference metastasis propensity for the eye, adrenal gland, ovary, and bone marrow. Because increased metastatic incidence for these organs and growth was shown in selected sublines in our experiments, it is likely that certain factor(s) common to these organs influence the metastatic preference of these cell lines. We assume that sensitivity of these cells is related to steroid hormone receptors, but elucidation of this hypothesis must await further studies.

Chapter V

FURTHER INVESTIGATIONS REQUIRED FOR MOLECULAR DETERMINANTS IN ORGAN PREFERENCE METASTASIS

Recent advances in genomic technology enable the transfection of animals/cells by certain genomes but also the creation of animals/cells lacking certain genes (knock-out animals), and these animals/cells play an important role in researching organ preference metastasis [53, 54]. Experiments using transplantable tumor lines can demonstrate precise results for organ preference metastasis-related molecules with regard to growth factors, adhesion, chemotactic factors, and other parameters [55-66].

However, generalization of implications of these molecules is usually very difficult [67], with elucidation of their clinical application being required [1, 33].

We investigated the molecules, especially cell adhesion molecules including carbohydrates, in reference to tumor metastasis, using various types of human cancer and experimental tumors.

At present, we believe that organ preference metastasis cannot be explained by single molecules. This is expected, because organ preference metastasis is a feature that is composed of a linkage involving several organs (Figure 39).

The findings on molecular bases will be described in the following chapter. We would first like to describe the three aspects of our research for future clinical application of organ preference metastasis.

1. Origin and Differentiation of Tumor Cells

The histological type of malignant tumors should be determined as accurately as possible because the role of metastasis-related molecules is different from their histological origins. For example, sialyl-Lewis^X expression in colorectal cancer cells plays a key role in providing information on metastasis in patients with colonic adenocarcinoma but not in adenocarcinoma of the stomach (Section III) [68, 69].

Histological classification of malignant tumors is enormous. For example, "Tumours of the lung," in the World Health Organization's (WHO) *Classification of Tumors* [70] divides malignant epithelial tumor into eight types (squamous cell carcinoma, small cell carcinoma, adenocarcinoma, large cell carcinoma, adenosquamous carcinoma, sarcomatoid carcinoma, carcinoid tumor, and salivary gland tumor). In addition, some of them are subdivided into ten types, as in the case of adenocarcinoma: mixed subtype, acinar adenocarcinoma, papillary adenocarcinoma, bronchioloalveolar adenocarcinoma, solid adenocarcinoma, fetal adenocarcinoma, mucinous (colloid) adenocarcinoma, mucinous cystadenocarcinoma, signet-ring cell carcinoma, and clear cell adenocarcinoma.

2. Target Organ/Tissue

Organs usually consist of several types of tissues from both the functional and structural perspective. Tissues can be broadly divided into parenchymal cells and supporting cells: their proportion and form varies depending upon the organ in question. For example, brain metastases can localize in any of the four regions of the brain: meninges, parenchyma, choroid plexus, and ventricles.

It is evident that blood vessels hosting tumor cells greatly vary among tissues, as evidenced by the fact that blood vessels in the brain parenchyma demonstrate a blood–brain barrier (BBB), which rarely develops in blood vessels in the other three above-mentioned brain regions. It is also evident that the proliferation and growth of extravasated tumor cells markedly vary, suggesting that the mechanisms involved in metastasis are different. For example, there are at least four routes taken in lung metastasis: pulmonary arteries, bronchial arteries, lymphatics, and bronchi. Each type of metastasis has its own particular metastatic mechanism.

3. TNM Classification for Effective Applications

The TNM factor, according to the WHO [70], is effective in the evaluation of organ preference metastasis. In general, it could be claimed that evaluation of early cancer with regard to organ metastasis preference is impossible because tumor cells rarely metastasizes to distant organs. However, small cell carcinoma and certain types of neuroendocrine tumors metastasize to various organs/tissues even though these tumors are very small.

References

[1] Nguyen, DX; Bos, PD; Massague, J. Metastasis: from dissemination to organ-specific colonization. *Nature Rev. Cancer*, 2009, *9*, 274-284.

[2] Fidler, IJ. The pathogenesis of cancer metastasis: the "seed and soil" hypothesis revisited. *Nature Rev. Cancer*, 2003, *3*, 453-458.

[3] Kawaguchi, T. *Cancer metastasis: Theory and Its Clinical Application.* Tokyo: Kanehara; 1994. (in Japanese).

[4] Kawaguchi, T. *Fundamental Aspect of Cancer Metastasis.* Tokyo: Kanehara; 2002. (in Japanese).

[5] Kawaguchi, T. Cancer metastasis: characterization and identification of the behavior of metastatic tumor cells and the cell adhesion molecules, including carbohydrates. *Current Drug Targets Cardiovasc. Hematol. Dis.*, 2005, 5, 39 61.

[6] Kawaguchi, T; Saito, A. Pathology on organ preference cancer mctastasis. *Mebio*, 1992, *9*, 22-30. (in Japanese).

[7] Paget, S. The distribution of secondary growths in cancer of the breast. *Lancet*, 1889, *1*, 571-573.

[8] de la Monte, SM; Moore, GW; Hutchins, GM. Patterned distribution of metastases from malignant melanoma in humans. *Cancer Res.*, 1983, *43*, 3427-3433.

[9] Ewing, J. A treatise on tumors. In: *Neoplastic disease.* 3rd ed. Philadelphia: WB Saunders; 1928; 77-89.

[10] Walther, HE. Die Metastasen. In: *Krebsmetastasen.* Basel: Benno Schwarbe and Co.; 1948; 55-186.

[11] Viadana, E; Bross, IDJ; Pickren, JW. Cascade spread of blood-borne metastases in solid and nonsolid cancers of humans. In: Weiss L, Gilbert HA, editors. *Pulmonary Metastasis*. The Hague: Martinus Nijhoff; 1978; 142-167.

[12] Batson, OV. The vertebral vein system, Caldwell Lecture 1956. In: Weiss L, Gilbert HA, editors. *Bone Metastasis*. Boston: GK Hall; 1981; 21-48.

[13] Kawaguchi, T; Kawaguchi, M; Miners, KM; Lembo, TM; Nicolson, GL. Brain meninges tumor formation by in vivo-selected metastatic B16 melanoma variants in mice. *Clin. Expl. Metastasis*, 1983, *1*, 247-259.

[14] Kawaguchi, T; Ikeda, K. Experimental studies on factors affecting tumor in the liver I. A scrutiny of number of cells and volume of fluid inoculated. *Fukushima J. Med. Sci*., 1976, *23*, 11-16.

[15] Sugino, T; Kawaguchi, T. New metastatic tumor model using cancer cell nest from C3H mammary carcinoma. *Nyugan Kisokenkyu*, 1992, 2, 34-38. (in Japanese).

[16] Sato, H; Suzuki, M. Deformability and viability of tumor cells by transcapillary passage, with reference to organ affinity of metastasis in cancer. In: Weiss L, editor. *Fundamental Aspect of Metastasis*, Amsterdam: North-Holland; 1976; 311-317.

[17] Zeidman, I; Buss, JM. Transpulmonary passage of tumor cell emboli. *Cancer Res.*, 1952, 12, 731-733.

[18] Coman, DR; deLong, RP; MccUtcheon, M. Studies on the mechanisms of metastasis; the distribution of tumors in various organs in relation to the distribution of arterial emboli. *Cancer Res.*, 1951, 11, 648-651.

[19] Suzuki, M. Studies on metastasis XXIV. Experiments on the brain metastasis of the rat ascites hepatoma cells. *J. Tuberculosis and Leprosy*, 1968, 20, 181-194. (in Japanese).

[20] Asahina, S. Experimental studies on relationship between tumors and organs by direct transplantation of small number of cells of ascites tumor into tissues. *Fukushima Igaku Zasshi,* 1967, 17, 65-89. (in Japanese).

[21] Kawaguchi, T; Nakamura, K. Relationship between transcerebral passage of tumor cells and brain metastasis. *Gann,* 1977, 68, 65-71.

[22] Warren, BA. Arrest and extravasation of cancer cells with special reference to brain metastasis and microinjury hypothesis. In: Weiss L, Gilbert HA, Posner JB, editors. *Brain metastasis*, Boston: GK Hall; 1980; 81-99.

[23] Kobayashi, T; Kitamura, H; Tobai, S; Asahina, S; Nakamura, K. Experimental studies on hematogenous metastasis in the kidney(1) - effect of ischemia-. *Fukushima Igaku Zasshi*, 1980, 29, 247-257. (in Japanese).

[24] Endo, M. Effect of dead cell embolism on formation of haematogenous metastases in the brain. *Fukushima Igaku Zasshi,* 1980, 30, 189-203. (in Japanese).

[25] Kawaguchi, T; Kitamura, H; Nakamura, K. Tumor formation of rat ascites hepatoma cells in the traumatized brain. *Gann.*, 1979, 70, 337-342.

[26] Nakashima, Y; Kawaguchi, T; Nakamura, K. The mechanisms of metastasis formation in injured parietal peritoneum by Yoshida sarcoma cells: an electron microscopic study. *Fukushima J. Med. Sci.*, 1985, 31, 17-28.

[27] French, JE; Macfarlane, RG. *Hemostasis and thrombosis*. In: Florey HW, editor. General Pathology, London: Lloyd-Luke LTD; 1970; 273-317.

[28] Folkman, J. Tumor angiogenesis. *Adv. Cancer Res.*, 1985, 43, 175-203.

[29] Dvorak, HF. Tumors: wounds that do not heal. Similarities between tumor stroma generation and wound healing. *N. Engl. J. Med.*, 1986, 315, 1650-1659.

[30] Kraft, KP. Tissue repair: the hidden drama. *Organogenesis*, 2010, 6, 225-233.

[31] Orr, FW; Warner, DJ. Effects of systemic complement activation and neutrophil-mediated pulmonary injury on the retention and metastasis of circulating cancer cells in mouse lungs. *Lab. Invest.*, 1990, 62, 331-338.

[32] Soares, FA; Shaughnessy, SG; MacLarkey, WR; Orr, FW. Quantification and morphologic demonstration of reactive oxygen species produced by Walker 256 tumor cells in vitro and during metastasis in vivo. *Lab. Invest.*, 1994, 71, 480-489.

[33] Dinarello, CA; Why not treat human cancer with interleukin-1 blockade? *Cancer Metastasis Rev.*, 2010, 29, 317-329.

[34] Poste, G. Experimental systems for analysis of the malignant phenotype. *Cancer Metastasis Rev.*, 1982, 1, 141-199.

[35] Nicolson, GL. Cancer metastasis: tumor cell and host organ properties important in metastasis to specific secondary sites. *Biochim. Biophys. Acta*, 1988, 948, 175-224.

[36] Matsuura, N; Puzon-McLaughlin, W; Irie, A; Morikawa, Y; Kakudo, K; Takada, Y. Induction of experimental bone metastasis in mice by transfection of integrin α4β1 into tumor cells. *Am. J. Pathol.*, 1996, 148, 55-61.
[37] Odashima, S. Establishment of ascites hepatomas in the rat, 1951-1962. *J. Natl. Cancer Inst. Monogr.*, 1964, 16, 51-93.
[38] Isaka, H; Satoh, H; Hirai, H. Variants of Yoshida ascites hepatoma and α-feto protein. In: NakaharaW, Ono T, Sugimura T, editors. *Differentiation and control of malignancy of tumor cells.* Tokyo: Univ. of Tokyo Press; 1974; 311-323.
[39] Sato, H. Experimental pathological studies on the metastasis of ascites tumors. *Nihon Byori Gakkai Kaishi*, 1967, 56, 9-36. (in Japanese).
[40] Kawaguchi, T. Experimental studies on transcerebral passage of tumor cells and formation of brain metastasis. *Fukushima Igaku Zasshi*, 1975, 24, 45-54. (in Japanese).
[41] Kawaguchi, T; Endo, M; Yokoya, S; Nakamura, K. Influence of lodgement site on the proliferation–kinetics of tumor cells. *Experientia*, 1981, 37, 414-415.
[42] Kawaguchi, T; Endo, M; Yokoya, S; Nakamura, K. Difference in proliferation–kinetics between tumor cells arrested in the brain and liver. *Experientia*, 1982, 38, 1236-1237.
[43] Kawaguchi, T; Nakamura, K. Analysis of the lodgement and extravasation of tumor cells in experimental models of hematogenous metastasis. *Cancer Metastasis Rev.*, 1986, 5, 77-94.
[44] Sato, Y. A thesis. Fukushima Medical University School of Medicine, No.230, (in Japanese).
[45] Fidler, IJ. Selection of successive tumour lines for metastasis. *Nat. New Biol.*, 1973, 242, 148-149.
[46] Brunson, KW; Beattie, G; Nicolson, GL. Selection and altered properties of brain-colonising metastatic melanoma. *Nature*, 1978, 272, 543-545.
[47] Nicolson, GL; Custead, SE. Tumor metastasis is not due to adaptation of cells to a new organ environment. *Science*, 1982, 215, 176-178.
[48] Kawaguchi, T; Kawaguchi, M; Lembo, TM; Nicolson, GL. Differential tumor growth of blood-borne B16 melanoma variants in cerebral dura mater is related to tumor-host cell reactions. *Clin. Exp. Metastasis*, 1989, 7, 1-14.
[49] Nicolson, GL; Menter, DG. Trophic factors and central nervous system metastasis. *Cancer Metastasis Rev.*, 1995, 14, 303-321.

[50] Watanabe, K. Experimental study on organ preference on cancer metastasis: establishment and characterization of highly metastatic sublines to eye ball derived from rat ascites hepatoma AH7974. *Fukushima Igaku Zasshi*, 1989, 39, 575-584. (in Japanese).

[51] Saito, A. The development of useful experimental model for analysis of organ preference on cancer metastasis: the establishment of highly metastatic cell lines to rat ovary and their metastatic propensity. *Fukushima Igaku Zasshi*, 1989, 39, 585-595. (in Japanese).

[52] Hoshi, N. Establishment of highly metastatic subline Bo-4 from rat ascites hepatoma AH7974. (A thesis. Fukushima Medical University School of Medicine, No. 200, 1995, in Japanese).

[53] Mundy, GR. Metastasis to bone: causes, consequences and therapeutic opportunities. *Nat. Rev. Cancer*, 2002, 2, 584-593.

[54] Mehta, HH; Gao, Q; Galet, C; Paharkova, V; Wan, J; Said, J; Sohn, JJ; Lawson, G; Cohen, P; Cobb, LJ; Lee, KW. IGFBP-3 is a metastasis suppression gene in prostate cancer. *Cancer Res.*, 2011, 71, 5154-5163.

[55] Ibrahim, T; Leong, I; Sanchez-Sweatman, O; Khokha, R; Sodek, J; Tenenbaum, HC; Ganss, B; Cheifetz, S. Expression of bone sialoprotein and osteopontin in breast cancer bone metastases. *Clin. Exp. Metastasis*, 2000, 18, 253-260.

[56] Müller, A; Homey, B; Soto, H; Ge, N; Catron, D; Buchanan, ME; McClanahan, T; Murphy, E; Yuan, W; Wagner, SN; Barrera, JL; Mohar, A; Verásteguim, E; Zlotnik, A. Involvement of chemokine receptors in breast cancer metastasis. *Nature*, 2001, 410, 50-56.

[57] Kang, Y; Siegel, PM; Shu, W; Drobnjak, M; Kakonen, SM; Cordón-Cardo, C; Guise, TA; Massagué, J. A multigenic program mediating breast cancer metastasis to bone. *Cancer Cell*, 2003, 3, 537-549.

[58] Lehr, JE; Pienta, KJ. Preferential adhesion of prostate cancer cells to a human bone marrow endothelial cell line. *J. Natl. Cancer Inst.*, 1998, 90, 118-123.

[59] Barthel, SR; Wiese, GK; Cho, J; Opperman, MJ; Hays, DL; Siddiqui, J; Pienta, KJ; Furie, B; Dimitroff, CJ. Alpha 1,3 fucosyltransferases are master regulators of prostate cancer cell trafficking. *Proc. Natl. Acad. Sci. USA*, 2009, 106, 19491-19496.

[60] Uehara, H; Kim, SJ; Karashima, T; Shepherd, DL; Fan, D; Tsan, R; Killion, JJ; Logothetis, C; Mathew, P; Fidler, IJ. Effects of blocking platelet-derived growth factor-receptor signaling in a mouse model of experimental prostate cancer bone metastases. *J. Natl. Cancer Inst.*, 2003, 95, 458-470.

[61] Diamond, JR; Finlayson, CA; Borges, VF. Hepatic complications of breast cancer. *Lancet Oncol.*, 2009, 10, 615-621.

[62] Sato, M; Narita, T; Kimura, N; Zenita, K; Hashimoto, T; Manabe, T; Kannagi, R. The association of sialyl Lewis(a) antigen with the metastatic potential of human colon cancer cells. *Anticancer Res.*, 1997, 17, 3505-3511.

[63] Brodt, P; Fallavollita, L; Bresalier, RS; Meterissian, S; Norton, CR; Wolitzky, BA. Liver endothelial E-selectin mediates carcinoma cell adhesion and promotes liver metastasis. *Int. J. Cancer*, 1997, 71, 612-619.

[64] Langley, RR; Fidler, IJ. The seed and soil hypothesis revisited- the role of tumor–stroma interactions in metastasis to different organs. *Int. J. Cancer*, 2011, 128, 2527-2535.

[65] Kaplan, RN; Rafii, S; Lyden, D. Preparing the "soil": the premetastatic niche. *Cancer Res.*, 2006, 66, 11089-11093.

[66] Hiratsuka, S; Watanabe, A; Aburatani, H; Maru, Y. Tumour-mediated upregulation of chemoattractants and recruitment of myeloid cells predetermines lung metastasis. *Nat. Cell Biol.*, 2006, 8, 1369-1375.

[67] Zeamari, S; Roos, E; Stewart, FA. Tumour seeding in peritoneal wound sites in relation to growth-factor expression in early granulation tissue. *Eur. J. Cancer*, 2004, 40, 1431-1440.

[68] Takano, Y; Teranishi, Y; Terashima, S; Motoki, R; Kawaguchi, T. Lymph node metastasis-related carbohydrate epitopes of gastric cancer with submucosal invasion. *Surg. Today*, 2000, 30, 1073-1082.

[69] Konno, A; Hoshino, Y; Terashima, S; Motoki, R; Kawaguchi, T. Carbohydrate expression profile of colorectal cancer cells is relevant to metastatic pattern and prognosis. *Clin. Exp. Metastasis*, 2002, 19, 61-70.

[70] World Health Organization Classification of Tumours, *Pathology and Genetics: Tumours of the lung, pleura, thymus and heart*. Travis WD, Brambilla E, Muller-Hermelink HK, Harris CC, editors. Lyon: IARCPress; 2004.

SECTION 3

METASTATIC POTENTIAL

SUMMARY AND CONCLUSION

Malignant tumors have the power to kill the host. It is apparent that invasion and metastasis, especially metastasis, are main agents. All malignant tumors have different metastatic potential, and the related factors can be divided approximately into the following three categories: 1) clinical/pathological, 2) cellular/biological, and 3) molecular/biochemical. Among them, we are especially interested in tumor cell-substrate adhesiveness and developed a new experimental model where the relationship between substrate adhesiveness and metastatic potential of tumor cells is evaluated. The results indicated that highly metastatic tumor cells have 62 and 54~56 kDa laminin-like substance with GS-I-B4 lectin-binding carbohydrates {terminal α-Galactose (α-Gal) residues}, and actually pretreatment of highly metastatic tumor cells with anti-laminin (LN) antibody or with human blood group A serum (containing natural antibody to the α-Gal-containing epitope) dramatically reduced the lung-colonizing potential of the cells.

Concerning metastatic potential of human cancers, our studies suggest that metastatic potential of tumors is intimately associated with the interaction of tumor cells and host tissues, especially with respect to cell surface adhesion molecules including carbohydrates. Preliminary examinations on expression of fibronectin (FN), LN, type IV collagen (CL-IV), and heparan sulphate proteoglycans (HSPGs) generated very limited insight. In contrast, examination of carbohydrates led us to new areas of investigation. Thus, we focused our studies on the relationship between carbohydrate expression by malignant tumor cells in primary sites and metastatic potential. We confirmed that tumor cell carbohydrate expression in malignant tumors is significantly related to ly and v factors, metastasis, and prognosis. For example, overexpression of fucosylated carbohydrate recognized by Le^x, SLe^{x-i}, and SLe^a was related to venous invasion and liver metastasis.

It is well known that SLe^a and SLe^x antigens are ligands of the selectin family, especially E-selectin, which is expressed on activated endothelial cells in tiny blood vessels around colorectal cancer tissues and metastatic foci in the liver. In contrast, overexpression of galactose/*N*-acethyl galactosamine (Gal/GalNAc) residues is related to-lymphatic vessel invasion and lymph node metastasis.

The carbohydrates expressed by tumor cells have received much attention as molecules related to metastasis and prognosis. However, the relationship is not as strong as expected. We believe that metastatic processes occur fundamentally through molecular interactions, but metastasis-related pathological phenomena are too complex to be explained only as related to individual carbohydrates. Each step apparently involves numerous molecular assemblies, and several kinds of tumor cell carbohydrates are used in each assembly.

We examined the relationship between carbohydrate expression of tumor cells in primary lesions and lymph node metastasis of breast cancer through analysis of the relationship between carbohydrate expression as recognized by two kinds of lectins and/or monoclonal antibodies (MAbs) and lymph node metastasis status. We found that 31 combinations of two lectins and/or MAbs correlated significantly with lymph node metastasis. Single lectins and MAbs, however, rarely correlate with lymph node metastasis. These combinations form a completely interrelated linkage (or network), when all lectins and MAbs in the combinations are connected with one another. The network included linkages among anti-Tn, *Vicia villosa agglutinin* (VVA), anti-human blood group H (anti-H), *Anguilla angulla* lectin (AAA), and anti-Le^x in the center; VVA occupied the central core, which may be due to VVAs being the only reagent among them significantly related to lymphatic invasion (ly factor).

We continue to study the carbohydrate epitope and molecules having VVA-binding carbohydrates in human breast cancer and rat ascites hepatoma AH109A cells that metastasize preferentially to lymph nodes. Results have shown that VVA recognizes the GalNAc residue of ~33 kDa MUC1 glycoprotein in tumor cells, which resembles Tn antigen {GalNAcα1-O-serine/threonin (Ser/Thr)}, but the precise molecular structure must await further studies.

INTRODUCTION

Malignant tumors have the power to kill the host when no effective treatment is given. Even when appropriate treatment is provided, malignant tumors may overwhelm the host, resulting in death because of infection, hemorrhagic disorder, so-called cachexia, or many other factors. Although invasion and metastasis are not solely responsible for the death of the host, it is apparent that these can be the main agents, especially metastasis. All malignant tumors have different metastatic potential. In addition, as described in detail in Section 1, metastatic formation is based on either the tumor cells themselves or stroma, including the so-called niche, or both. Therefore, there are numerous factors associated with metastatic potential. Here, we briefly summarize the current theory on metastatic potential of tumor cells, and then describe our own investigations on the role of adhesion molecules and carbohydrates using human materials and experimental systems.

Chapter VI

FACTORS RELATED TO METASTATIC POTENTIAL OF TUMOR CELLS

We consider that factors involved in metastatic potential of tumor cells can be divided approximately into the following three categories: (1) clinical/pathological, (2) cellular/biological, and (3) molecular/biochemical (Table 9). No distinct demarcation lines exist among these.

1. CLINICAL/PATHOLOGICAL FACTORS

This category includes diverse factors such as age, gender, race, area of residence, nutritional state, and performance status. Age is known to be a potential metastatic factor, as seen in case of gastric cancer, where the condition is more aggressive in younger patients [1]. Gender is an important factor in prognosis of several malignant tumors, including melanoma [2]. The macroscopic appearance of a tumor (including color) is useful for evaluating its aggressive character. Figure 46 shows a case of inflammatory breast cancer with irregular red coloration of the skin, a hallmark of severe lymphatic invasion by breast cancer. Bormann's type IV gastric cancer frequently metastasizes to the coelomic cavity, resulting in poor prognosis. Size and depth of invasion are included in the World Health Organization's (WHO) tumor staging of tumor development.

Histologically, several tumor types may be correlated with metastatic potential [3]. For example, small cell carcinoma of the lung is highly metastatic, and patient prognosis is poor (Figure 47).

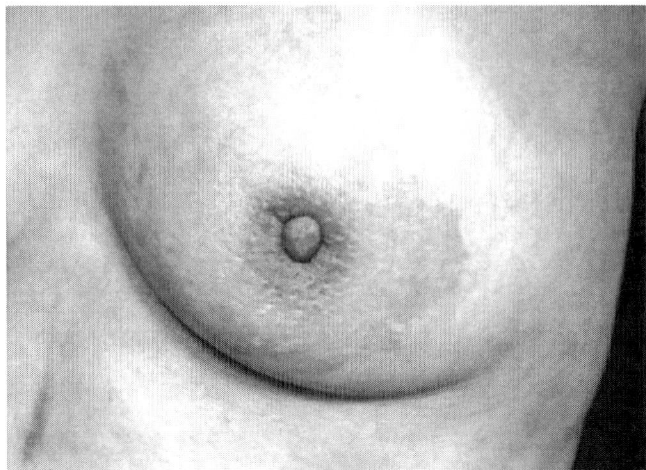

Figure 46. Inflammatory breast cancer. This type of breast cancer rarely forms a distinct tumor mass. Tumor cells invaded aggressively into lymphatic vessels and metastasized to lymph nodes.

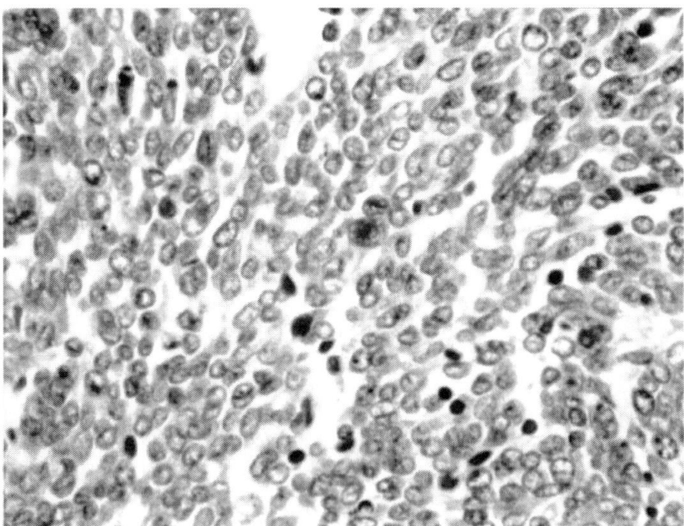

Figure 47. Small cell carcinoma of the lung. There are four representative histological types of lung cancer: squamous cell carcinoma, adenocarcinoma, small cell carcinoma, and large cell carcinoma. Small cell carcinoma of the lung expresses neuroendocrine markers such as chromogranin, synaptophysin, and/or CD56. This tumor frequently metastasizes to various organs, especially the liver and the brain, even though they may be small in size.

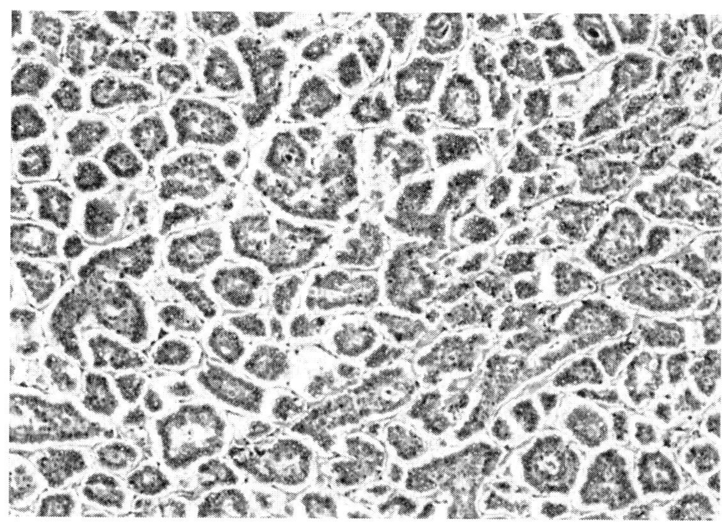

Figure 48. Micropapillary carcinoma of the breast. This type of breast cancer is highly metastatic. We consider that cell surface MUC1 is associated with its cellular behavior.

Neuroendocrine tumors have high metastatic potential, as micropapillary carcinoma of the breast (Figure 48), the uterus, and other sites do [4]. In contrast, basal cell carcinoma of the skin rarely metastasizes, although there is marked local invasion. The degree of differentiation of tumor cells is another hallmark of metastatic potential. In general, poorly differentiated tumors appear to possess higher metastatic potential than well-differentiated ones. Atypia, both cellular and structural, is also useful for predicting metastatic potential. In these cases, pathologists may evaluate metastatic potential of tumors from the standpoint of tumor progression.

Proliferation of and necrosis caused by malignant tumors sometimes reflects their metastatic potential [3]. These factors may not only be associated with tumor cells themselves but also reflect tumor vessel density; in fact, there is a positive correlation between tumor blood vessel density and metastatic potential [5]. This leads to the increased likelihood of intravasation of tumor cells.

Changes in the interstitium of tissues, especially displacement by fibrocytes, fibroblasts, and/or myofibroblasts (dysmoplasia), are seen frequently in several types of malignant tumors and are related to their metastatic potential (Figure 49) [6]. At present, precise mechanisms involved in tumor sclerosis are unknown, but poor blood supply causes tumor cell anoxia followed by enhancement of metastatic potential.

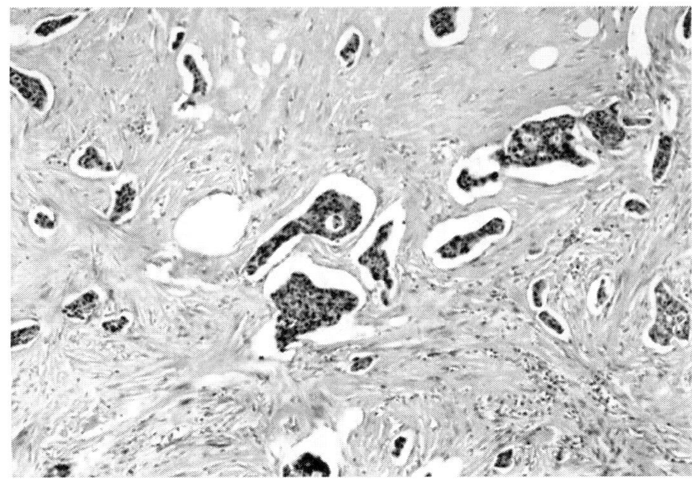

Figure 49. Scirrhous carcinoma of the breast. Carcinoma cells invade into fibrous tissue with mild lymphocytic infiltration.

Levels of intravasation (v factor) and intralymphatic vessel invasion (ly factor) should be determined under preparations stained by CD31 or D2-40 antibodies, respectively, because it is generally difficult to distinguish blood vessels and lymphatic vessels. For determination of intravasation by tumor cells in larger blood vessels such as veins, we utilize preparations stained with elastica–Masson (Figure 15). Metastasis in lymph node, organ, and/or coelomic cavity is directly related to prognosis, although recent advances in therapy have improved prognosis in certain cases.

2. Cellular/Biological Factors

Motility, floating, *in vitro* cultivation, and transplantability of tumor cells are considered to be cellular and/or biological factors. We are of the opinion that cellular motility should be mentioned here because tumor cell motility in culture cannot be evaluated accurately in quantitative molecular terms [7, 8]. Floating of tumor cells is inherent in the process of metastasis, and therefore metastatic tumor cells have to acquire some degree of floating ability [9]. Indeed, tumor cells that acquire the ability to float are more metastatic than substrate-dependent cells, but the converse is not true (see next section of this chapter) [10, 11]. *In vitro* growth of human tumor cells has been reported to be correlated with metastatic potential [12].

Table 9. Factors affecting metastatic potential/malignancy of tumors

1. Clinical/pathological factors
· Age, gender, race, resident area, nutrition state, performance status, and others
· Gross appearance
· Location
· Size and depth of invasion
· Histological type
· Proliferating index
· Necrosis
· Vascular density
· Fibrosis
· Vascular invasion {lymphatic vessel invasion (ly) factor, blood vessel invasion (v) factor}, and neural invasion (neu/pn) factor}
2. Biological factors
· Cellular mobility
· Floating ability in culture
· In vitro cultivation
· Transplantation ability in nude mice
3. Molecular factors
· Growth factor/growth factor receptor
· Adhesion molecule/carbohydrate
· Chemotaxis/motility factor
· Protease/protease inhibitor
· Coagulation/fibrinolysis
· Host defense mechanism
· Chromosome, oncogene, suppressor gene, chromosome number, DNA, ploidy

3. Molecular/Biochemical Factors

Epidermal growth factor (EGF) and EGF-receptor (EGF-R) are involved in the regulation of growth and differentiation of many types of cells [13]. EGF-R overexpression is known to be related to augmented metastatic potential and poor prognosis in many types of malignant tumors, including not only squamous cell carcinoma of esophagus, lung, uterine cervix, oral cavity, and skin, but also in other types of malignant tumors such as adenocarcinoma and malignant mesenchymal tumors [14].

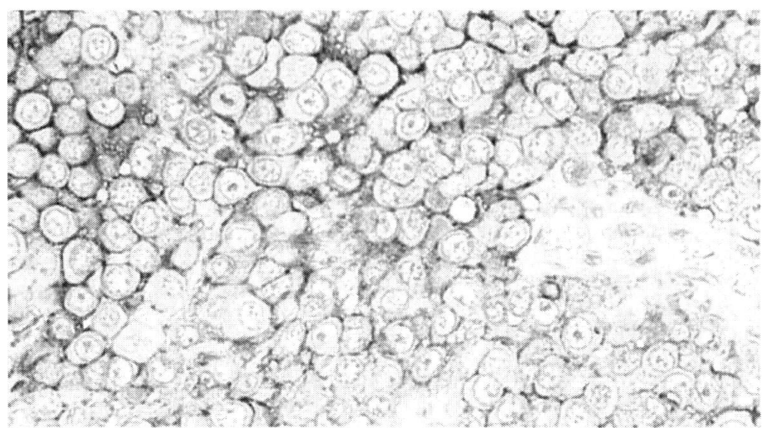

Figure 50. Immunohistochemical expression of HER2 antigen of breast cancer cells in metastatic brain tumor.

The mechanism by which tumor cells acquire high metastatic potential through EGF-R activation is suggested by altered and/or augmented production of integrins and extracellular matrix degradation enzymes [15]. The immunohistochemical degree of EGF-R and HER2 (Figure 50) by malignant tumors of breast, lung, stomach, and large intestine (cecum, colon and rectum) is currently estimated by pathologists to report clinicians.

There are many isoforms of TGF-β, collectively, forming a superfamily. TGF-β1 is a key molecule in human cells and is involved in suppression of cell proliferation; however, it has been demonstrated that many types of human cancers are not suppressed by TGF-β1. Contrastingly, several studies have demonstrated that TGF-β is associated with invasion and metastasis of tumor cells in the following ways: 1) inhibition of antitumor immunosuppressor activity, 2) enhancement of tumor cell motility, and 3) induction of tumor angiogenesis and fibroblast production [16]. Tumor cells produce various types of angiogenesis factors, such as acid FGF, angiogenin, basic FGF, heparinase, hepatocyte growth factor, interleukin-8, PDGF, pleiotrophin, prostaglandin E1, E2, TGF-α, TGF-β, tumor necrosis factor (TNF), and VEGF. VEGF is involved in development of blood and lymphatic vessels and contains VEGF-A, VEGF-B, VEGF-C, VEGF-D, VEGF-E, PIGF (placenta growth factor)-1, and PIGF-2. VEGF has strong angiogenetic activity, and its expression by tumor cells is correlated with metastatic potential [17].

Numerous cell locomotion/motility factors influence metastatic potential of tumor cells through autocrine and/or paracrine pathways. HGF is a scatter factor (SF) for epithelial cells, and its ligand is c-met; expression of HGF/SF and c-met is known to promote metastatic potential of tumor cells [18]. AMF/AMFR was isolated from a culture medium of human melanoma [19, 20]. It was demonstrated that binding of AMF to its receptor induced signal transduction, similar to chemotactic stimulation of neutrophil mobility, as well as the internalization and transport of its receptor to the leading edge, stimulating pseudopodial protrusion and cell motility. Tumor cell autocrine motility factor is the neuroleukin/phosphohexose isomerase polypeptide, whose serum value is used clinically as a tumor marker and is correlated positively to metastasis. More than 100 types of molecules belong to the Ras superfamily, divided into five subfamilies: Ras, Rho, Rab, Arf, and Ran. These families are known to be related to the metastatic spread of malignant tumors [21].

It is also well known that tumor cells frequently metastasize to granulation tissue, and, in turn, tumor cells in granulation tissue readily metastasize. Several workers have suggested that superoxide promotes tumor cell motility, resulting in metastasis [22]. Protease/protease inhibitors are key players in metastatic potential of tumor cells, and the biological/pathological significance of these is described in Chapter I. Briefly, in 1980, Liotta et al. [23] reported the relationship between type IV collagen degradation ability and lung metastatic potential of tumor cells. Subsequently, Nakajima et al. [24] reported the relationship between heparitinase production and lung metastatic potential of tumor cells. Since these pioneering studies, protease and protease inhibitor (TIMP) have been studied extensively in relation to invasion and metastasis of tumor cells. For a long time, coagulation, anticoagulation and fibrinolysis of tumor cells have been considered to be related to their metastatic potential, and several authors have indicated that anticoagulation drugs inhibit blood-borne metastasis [25]. More recent work supports the significance of an abnormal blood coagulation system in blood-borne metastasis [26]. The host defense mechanism and its related factors have been considered to be related closely to metastatic potential of some types of tumor cells [27]. This mechanism can be mediated not only by the classical tumor-specific antigen–antibody reaction but may also involve the autocrine/paracrine system of cytokines. The latter system may be related to metastatic potential of tumor cells but also to organ preference with regard to metastasis. Signal transfer networks are suspected to link other types of cell character such as adhesion, locomotion, and growth. In addition, natural killer cells and cytotoxic T cells are believed to destroy metastatic tumor cells [28, 29].

Several researchers have reported that augmented metastatic potential of tumors is correlated with irregular distribution of chromosomes and/or DNA aneuploidy. However, such correlation cannot be generalized, as previously described and shown in Figure 51. Some workers have reported on the relationship between augmented AgNOR expression by tumor cells and prognosis/metastasis, but others were unable to discern such a relationship. Cases of esophageal cancer with co-amplification of hst-1 and int-2 had poor prognosis with distant hematogenous metastasis [30]. This was predictable because these genes belong to the FGF family. Overexpression of cyclin D1 gene is also related to poor prognosis in esophageal cancer patients with distant metastasis [31], but the mechanism involved remains unknown. K-sam gene is amplified in scirrhous carcinoma of the stomach. This gene codes HGF-R and c-met, suggesting that its amplification relates to invasion and metastasis of tumor cells [32]. Point mutation of K-ras was found in greater than 90% cases of pancreatic cancer and 40%–50% cases of colorectal cancer, but there was no apparent relationship between K-ras mutation and metastasis in colorectal cancer [33, 34]. Amplifications of c-myc and N-myc genes, whose products are transcription factors, are correlated to invasion and metastasis of small cell carcinoma of the lung and neuroblastoma [35]. Amplification of fos, which was observed in squamous cell carcinoma and melanoma, is associated with augmented catepsin secretion and cell mobility [36].

We are currently investigating tumor suppressor gene protein p53, because we found a positive correlation between p53 expression and lymph node metastasis in both lung and gastric cancer. Furthermore, no correlation was found in hematogenous metastasis [37-39]. Therefore, it is important to elucidate how p53 mutation is related to lymph node metastasis. Our results indicate that p53 expression of tumor cells is positively correlated with expression of their Tn antigen and VVA carbohydrate antigen. Relationships between lymph node metastasis and Tn/VVA carbohydrate antigens will be discussed in the next chapter.

KAI1, a metastasis suppressor gene product, is a membrane glycoprotein that is a member of the transmembrane 4 superfamily. Expression of this gene has been shown to be down-regulated in tumor progression in human cancers and can be activated by p53 through a consensus binding sequence in the promoter. Its expression and expression of p53 are strongly correlated, and the loss of expression of these two proteins is associated with poor survival for prostate cancer patients [40]. p16 gene product is an inhibitor of cyclin-dependent kinase (CDK4). Defects or reduced expression of this product are correlated with metastasis in oral squamous cell carcinoma, esophageal squamous cell carcinoma, and melanoma [41]. Nm23 was isolated from a highly metastatic mouse melanoma [42]. This is a suppressor oncogene that encodes nucleoside diphosphate (NDP) kinase, and there are three types of relationships with regard to its expression level and metastatic potential: inverted correlation, positive correlation, and absence of correlation [43]. Inverted correlation was found in breast cancer, hepatocellular carcinoma, gastric cancer, and melanoma. Positive correlation was found in colorectal cancer, pancreatic cancer, and neuroblastoma. Absence of correlation was found in adenocarcinoma of the lung. The mechanism is still unclear, although a tumor cell–substrate adhesion mechanism is involved.

Mts-1 codes S100A4 protein and regulates cell motility and invasion [44]. Tiam1 is a GDP-dissociation stimulator (GDS) protein for Rho-like GTPases *in vitro*. In fibroblasts, Tiam1 induces a similar phenotype as constitutively activated (V12) Rac1, including membrane ruffling, and this is inhibited by the dominant (N17) Rac1. Moreover, T-lymphoma cells expressing V12 Rac1 become invasive, indicating that the Tiam1–Rac signaling pathway could operate in the invasion and metastasis of tumor cells [45].

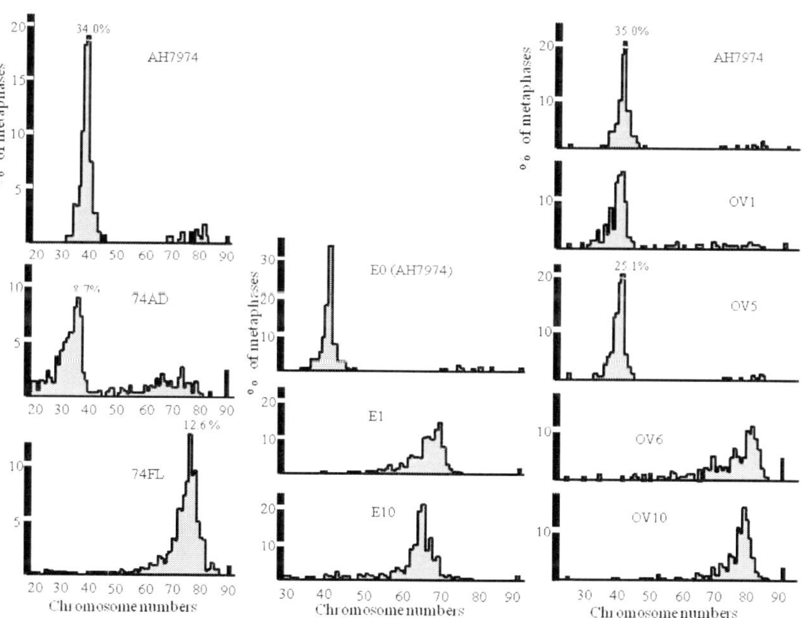

Figure 51. Variation in chromosome numbers of rat ascites hepatoma AH7974 variant sublines. See text for discussion of organ preference in metastasis [Section II, Reference 50-52].

Chapter VII

Identification and Characterization of Metastasis-Related Adhesion Molecules, with Special Reference to Extracellular Matrix (ECM) Proteins

Adhesion family includes families of cadherin (E-cadherin, N-cadherin, P-cadherin), Ig super family (ICAM-1, ICAM-2, VCAM-1, CD2, CD4, LFA-3), integrin family (β1 integrin: VLA-1, 2, 3, 4, 5, 6, β2 integrin: LFA-1, Mac-1, β3 integrin: gpIIb/IIIa, VNR), selectin family (L-, P-, and E-selectin), and others (CD44, PP addressin, PLN addressin). Although carbohydrates play various functions in addition to cellular adhesion, we include them in this group because recent studies suggest that carbohydrates are mainly related to metastasis via their function of cellular adhesion. We describe this in Section 3 in detail.

The altered adhesiveness of tumor cells to substrates has been linked to their metastatic properties. Extensive studies have attempted to define the elements associated with tumor cell substrate adhesiveness and to clarify their possible effects on metastasis [46, 47]. However, all but a few of these studies utilized tumor cells derived from transplantable solid tumors. We found two characteristics of the relationship between tumor cells and ECM in the natural history of tumor development and progression. First, tumor cells can acquire "growth capability while floating," and second, tumor cells inevitably float during the process of transport in metastasis (Chapter I). Klein [48] believed that anchorage-independent floating cells were produced by mutation and selection of solid tumor cells. In fact, Yoshida [49] succeeded in selecting ascites tumor sublines from solid tumor lines. With regard to the second characteristics, the capacity of tumor cells to float during the transport process in metastasis, Raz et al. [9] demonstrated that the metastasizing ability of tumor cells increases dramatically when substrate-adherent tumor cells are selected for their ability to float. However, little attention has been paid to the adhesion of floating tumor cells to substrates, especially with reference to cancer metastasis. The following text describes results from our studies of representative adhesion molecules.

1. Selection and Establishment of Adherent and Floating Cell Lines From Rat Ascites Hepatoma AH7974 and Their Metastatic Potential

When rat ascites hepatoma AH7974 cells were cultured in serum-supplemented medium, most cells floated. However, approximately 1 per 1,000 cells adhered to the culture dish. The adherent cells and the floating cells were then cultured separately. After the culture procedure was repeated several times, the adherent cell line 74AD and the floating cell line 74FL were established [Figure 52]. By a similar selection procedure, 74AD-f and 74FL-a were selected from 74AD and 74FL, respectively. Also, in order to study the ability of cells to produce ECM, we established cell lines with different substrate adhesion characteristics under serum-free conditions [10, 11, 50, 51]. 74AD and 74FL-a cells settled onto plastic, spread with prominent pseudopodia and finally grew into confluent monolayers with randomly arranged cells. Almost all 74AD-f and 74FL cells were suspended as single cells or small irregular cell clusters in culture medium; a few cells adhered to or were weakly attached to the culture plates (Figure 53).

The differences in chromosome numbers among AH7974, 74AD, and 74FL cells were obvious. The modal chromosome number of AH7974 cells was 42; more than 90% of the cells had a chromosome number approximately in the diploid range, and less than 5% had a number of the cells approximately in the triploid range. The modal chromosome numbers of 74AD and 74FL cells were 39 and 79, respectively, and both cell lines exhibited wide ranges in chromosome numbers. Giemsa-banding analysis revealed that the karyotypes of 74AD and 74FL cells were diploid and hyperdiploid, respectively, and that the difference in their chromosome numbers was caused by emergence within several minutes in 74FL cells. Large subtelocentric chromosomes, which were believed to originate from partial duplication of the long arm of chromosome No. 1, were often observed in 74FL cells. The marker chromosome of AH7974 was found in both variants, which indicates that the selected variants originated from the AH7974 line (Figure 51) [10].

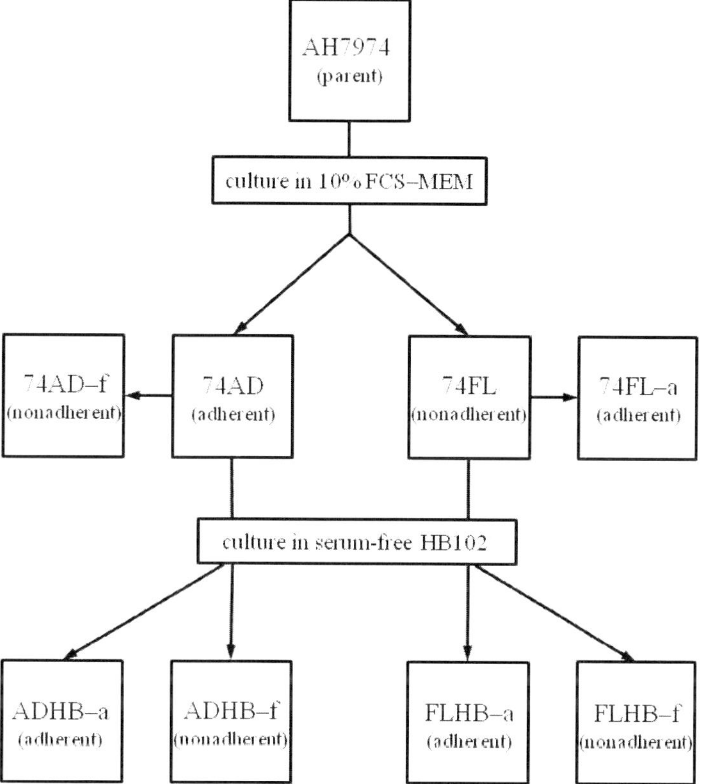

Figure 52. Selection and establishment of adherent and floating cell lines in serum-supplemented or serum-free medium. Rat ascites hepatoma AH7974 cells were cultured in minimum essential medium supplemented with 10% fetal calf serum (FCS-MEM). Most of the growing cells floated, but a few of them (less than 5%) adhered to and spread on the culture plates. The cell lines 74AD and 74FL were selected from adherent cells and floating cells by repeated selections, respectively. 74AD-f and 74FL-a were selected from 74AD and 74FL cells by repeated culture, respectively. Calcium-magnesium-free MEM was used for detachment of adherent cells. Similarly, ADHB-f and ADHB-a were selected from 74AD, and FLHB-f and FLHB-a were selected from 74FL. ADHB-f, ADHB-a, FLHB-a, and FLHB-f cell lines were cultured in serum-free HB102 medium [10, 11, 50, 51].

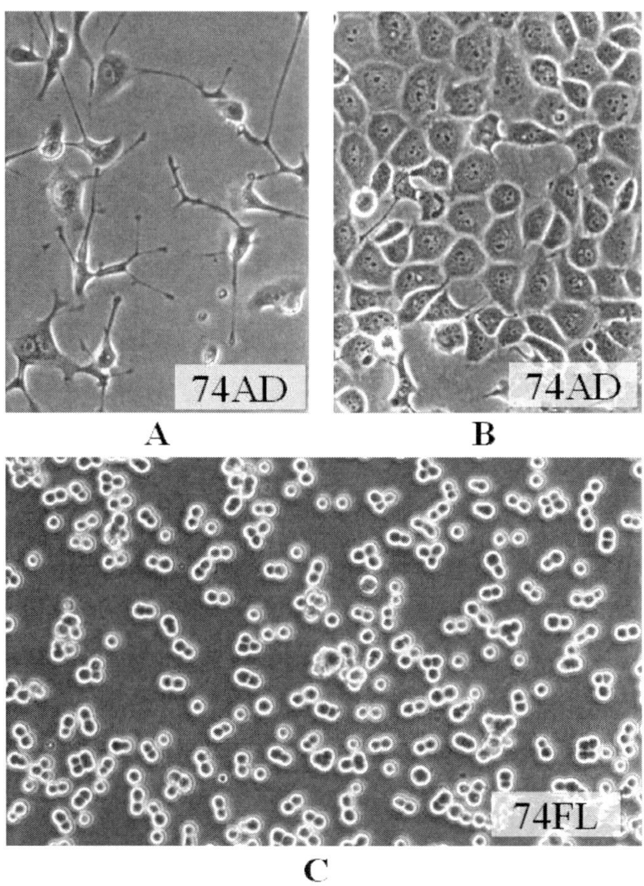

Figure 53. A: 74AD cells, after one day of culture, ×170. B: 74AD cells, after six days of culture, ×85. C: 74FL cells, after four days of culture, ×85. 74AD cells were seeded onto plastic, settled and spread with prominent pseudopodia, and finally grew into confluent monolayers with randomly arranged cells. 74FL cells developed as single suspended cells or small irregular cell clusters in culture medium. A few cells adhered to or were weakly attached to the culture plates [11].

2. Experimental Metastatic Potential of Rat Ascites Hepatoma AH7974 Sublines with Different Substrate Adhesiveness

After intravenous injection (10^6 cells/ml) into Donryu strain rats, 74AD, 74FL, and AH7974 cells yielded an average number of 183, 869 and 48 lung surface colonies, respectively; 74AD-f and 74FL-a cells showed low lung-colonizing abilities (fewer than ten lung colonies). Significant differences ($p<0.01$) were observed between the 74FL cells and the other 74AD, 74AD-f, and 74FL-a lines and between the 74AD cells and 74AD-f and 74FL-a cells. The metastasizing abilities of ADHB-a, ADHB-f, FLHB-a, and FLHB-f cells to the lung were not correlated with their substrate adhesiveness and were consistent with those of their precursor cell lines. The metastatic potentials of the ADHB-a and ADHB-f cell lines were lower than those of FLHB-a and FLHB-f. We therefore concluded that there was no obvious correlation between adhesiveness to the ECM in culture and lung metastatic potential of our cell lines [10, 11, 50, 51].

3. Minimum Essential Unit of Tumor Cell-ECM Adhesion Required for Lung Metastasis

74AD cells possessed high adhesion affinities for fibronectin (FN), laminin (LN), and type IV collagen (CL-IV). The cells also possessed a relatively high adhesion affinity to vitronectin (VN). In contrast, 74FL cells hardly adhered to these purified ECM proteins. The difference in *in vitro* adhesion between the two cell lines tended to increase after incubation of the cells in medium containing fetal bovine serum (Figure 54). 74AD and 74FL cells adhered avidly to the ECM of vascular endothelial cells, however, with 74AD cells adhering more rapidly than 74FL cells. Although 74AD cell-ECM adhesion was not inhibited by pretreatment of the ECM with anti-fibronectin (FN), anti-laminin (LN), or anti-type IV collagen (CL-IV) antibodies, it was considerably inhibited by pretreatment of the ECM with a mixture of these antibodies, especially with a combination of anti-FN and anti-LN [11].

From these results, we believe that 74FL cells lost the ability to adhere strongly to representative ECM proteins and glycosaminoglycans (GAGs), but they nevertheless had high metastatic potential to lung. ECM produced by vascular endothelial cells contained adhesion molecule(s) for tumor cells that had lost their ability to adhere strongly to isolated ECM proteins [11]. Thus, strong adhesion of tumor cells to the ECM is not crucial for metastasis to lung and, in fact, firm adhesion to the ECM may actually prevent the movement of tumor cells. Therefore, decreased but minimal adhesion appears to be advantageous for metastasis, and the highly metastatic 74FL cells have this minimal, essential capacity.

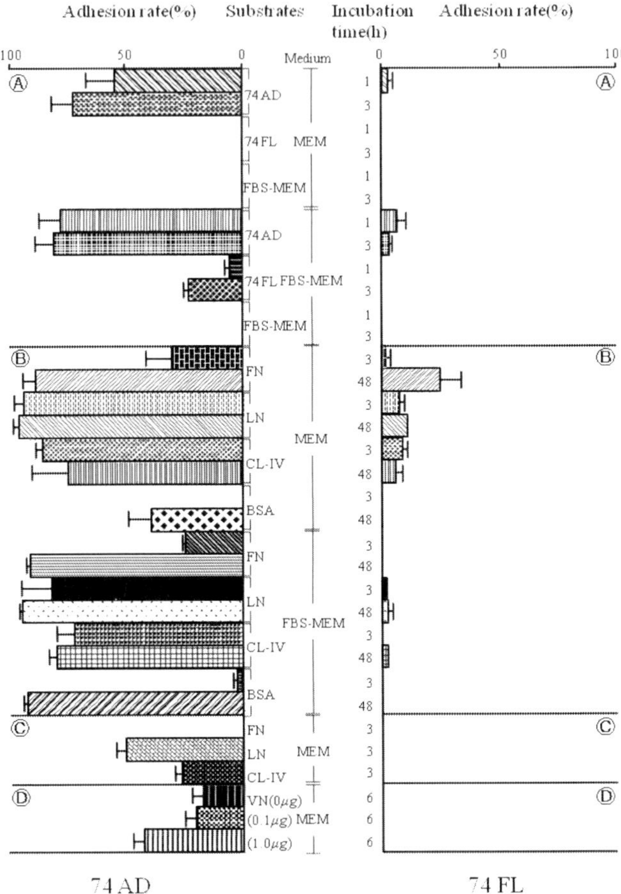

Figure 54. Adhesion characteristics of 74AD and 74FL cells under various culture conditions. (A) Adhesion to culture substrates. (B) Adhesion to purified ECM proteins. (C) Adhesion of trypsin-EDTA-treated cells to purified fibronectin (FN), laminin (LN) and type IV collagen (CL-IV). (D) Effect of vitronectin (VN) on adhesion of cells to plastic. BSA: bovine serum albumin; FBS: fetal bovine serum [11].

Our results are not consistent with those of some other workers, who have claimed that highly metastatic tumor cells possess a capacity for stronger adhesion ability to FN, LN, CL-IV, or ECM produced by vascular endothelial cells than do tumor cells with low metastatic potential, even when cells from the same parental strain were compared [52-54]. However, if metastatic potential is correlated with the degree of anaplasia of tumor cells in terms of extracellular adhesion molecule formation, there is no discrepancy between their results and ours.

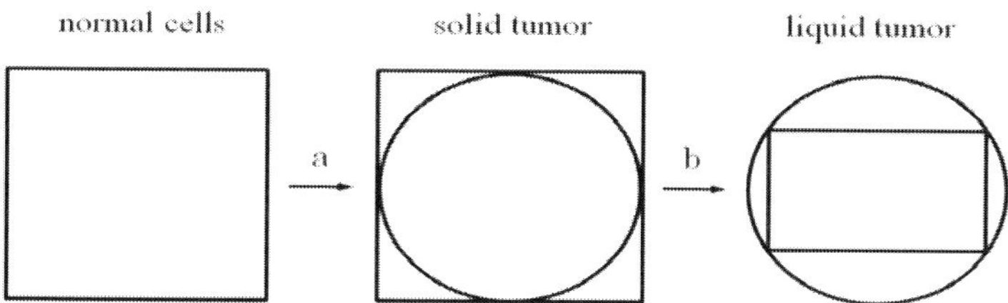

Figure 55. Relationships of untransformed (normal) cells, transplantable solid tumor cells, and transplantable liquid tumor cells to substrate adhesiveness. The square and circle show anchorage-dependence and anchorage-independence, respectively (a, malignant transformation; b, selection and mutation) [11]. This schematic suggests that an entire population of untransformed cells is anchorage-dependent and that cells from solid tumors are also fundamentally anchorage-dependent. Solid tumor cells are anchorage-independent under some conditions, and liquid tumor cells acquire anchorage-independence. Under certain conditions, liquid tumor cells can adhere to substrates, however. As anaplasia progresses, cells lose individual adhesion properties.

In this case, the most advanced anaplastic cells would be defined as those cells that have lost almost all adhesion to ECM components except for a minimal essential unit of adhesion (Figure 55).

We concluded that the quality rather than the strength of adhesion of metastatic tumor cells to ECM components is important. This characteristic allows the tumor cells to migrate to surrounding tissues after adhesion. The 67 kDa LN receptor (LNR) and VLA3, which were suggested to be related to metastasis of human cancers [46, 52], may be examples of molecules that permit such migration.

4. Production of ECM Components and Metastatic Potential

The relationship between the ability to synthesize ECM components and metastatic potential of tumor cells is another area of interest. Here, we describe our results with GAGs, FN, and LN.

4.1. Glycosaminoglycans (GAGs)

We examined and quantified the production and retention of GAGs by all cell line variants by using two-dimensional electrophoresis [55]. The amounts of GAGs did not differ among the cell lines, but marked differences were found in GAG distribution, especially of heparan sulfate (HS). In 74FL cell cultures, about 70% of the total HS was found in the culture medium in soluble form, whereas in 74AD cell cultures, only 7% was found in the medium, and the rest was in the cell-substrate complex. The increased HS in the culture medium of 74FL cells was apparently caused by failure of the cell surface to retain HS and not by increased production of the GAG.

Low levels of cell surface HS correlated with high metastatic activity of many tumors [56]. The experiment of Nakajima et al. [24] may shed some light on the effect of low levels of cell surface HS proteoglycans (HSPGs) of 74FL cells. They reported a correlation between HS degradation and lung metastatic potential of B16 melanoma variant sublines. Because cell surface HSPGs are thought to inhibit invasion by promoting tight cell-cell and cell-ECM adhesion, the reduced cell surface retention of HSPGs by 74FL cells would be advantageous for cells to be able to move.

4.2. Fibronectin (FN)

Cell surface FN was observed on the low metastatic potential cell line 74AD but disappeared almost completely from the cell line with high metastatic potential, 74FL [10]. Expression of cell surface fibronectin receptor (FNR) paralleled that of cell surface FN, but the total amount of FNR (GP125, [57]) estimated by Western blotting was much higher in 74FL cells than in 74AD cells [10]. Therefore, we believe that low expression of FNR on the cell surface is not due to an inability to produce it but to a failure of its expression on the cell surface. This idea seems to be supported by the observation of Rieber et al. [58], who found that a certain kind of FNR on the cell surface disappeared when B16 melanoma cells became spherical. In this situation, cell surface FN may be related to opsonin activity [59].

4.3. Laminin (LN)

The relationship between the expression of anti-LN antibody-binding protein (LN-like substance) and the metastatic potential of murine fibrosarcoma cells was first reported by Varani et al. [60]. They found that the LN-like substance had a molecular size of 56kDa and possessed an α-D-galactose (α-Gal) residue. We also found that rat ascites hepatoma AH7974 cells expressed on the cell surface LN-like substances and carbohydrate(s) {oligosaccharides containing α-Gal recognized by *Griffonia Bandeiraea simplicifolia* isolectin B4 (GS-I-B4)}[50]. Expression of α-Gal-containing oligosaccharide was apparently not influenced by pretreatment of cells with methanol. The cell membrane LN-like substances had approximate molecular sizes of 150, 62 and 54~56 kDa under denaturing and reducing conditions; the 62 and 54~56 kDa bands stained with GS-I-B4 (Figure 56). Therefore, the AH7974 cell membrane molecules bearing α-Gal-containing oligosaccharide residues were considered to be LN-like substances. All cell lines (74AD, 74AD-f, 74FL, 74FL-a) strongly expressed these LN-like molecules, but a marked difference was found in the expression of α-Gal-containing oligosaccharides, which were expressed most strongly by 74FL cells (30-50%), followed by 74AD cells (less than 10%), and rarely by 74AD-f cells (less than 1%) and 74FL-a cells (less than 0.1%).We also analyzed the expression of LN mRNA and LN- binding protein mRNA in these cell lines. The binding protein mRNA was expressed in all cell lines in almost equal amounts. LN A chain mRNA was absent in all cell lines; expression of LN B1 and LN B2 chain mRNAs differed among the cell lines [109].

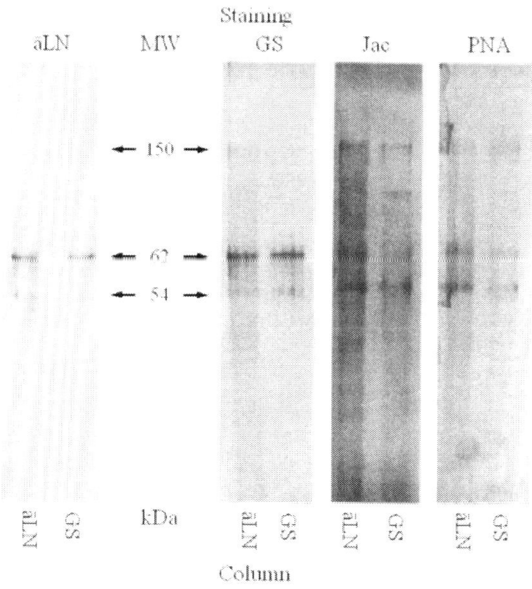

Figure 56. Western blotting analysis of cell membrane laminin (LN)-like substances and α-Gal-containing molecules of AH7974 cells. The cell membrane LN-like substances (aLN) and α-Gal-containing molecules were isolated by means of HPLC affinity chromatography with anti-LN antibody and GS-I-B4 (GS), respectively. These proteins were also reacted with Jacalin (Jac) and PNA [50].

4.4. Effects of Pretreatment of Tumor Cells by Anti-LN Antibody or by Human Type A Serum on Lung Metastatic Potential

Pretreatment of 74FL cells with anti-LN antibody or with human blood group type A serum (containing natural antibody to the α-Gal-containing oligosaccharide epitope) dramatically reduced the lung-colonizing potential of the cells [50].

Table 10. Augmentation of lung metastatic potential by culturing tumor cells with human serum of blood group type A

Cell line	Total number of animals used	Number of animals with lung metastasis	Average number of lung colonies	Average lung weight (g)
74AD				
H-0	10	9	40.9	1.65
H-5	10	8	122.8	1.86
H-10	5	1	0.2	1.44
74AD-f				
H-0	10	2	0.6	1.42
H-5	10	1	0.3	1.32
H-10	5	1	0.2	1.21
74FL				
H-0	20	19	161.4	1.91
H-5	10	8	Too many to count	4.43
H-10	5	5	Too many to count	4.09
74FL-a				
H-0	10	3	0.6	1.86
H-5	10	1	0.1	1.42
H-10	7	0	0.0	1.55

All ascites hepatoma AH7974 variant sublines (74AD, 74AD-f, 74FL, 74FL-a) strongly expressed anti-laminin (LN) antibody-reactive substance (laminin-like molecule), but α-Gal containing oligosaccharide recognized by GS-I-B4 was expressed to greatly different degrees among the cell lines, in the order 74FL>74AD>74FL-a=74AD-f. The degree of expression was in accordance with lung metastatic potential. To investigate the significance of carbohydrate expression, the cell lines were first cultured in minimal essential medium MEM supplemented with 10% fetal calf serum (FCS) and then in MEM supplemented with human blood group type A serum, which contains natural antibody to α-Gal, for five generations (H-5) and ten generations (H-10) [61].

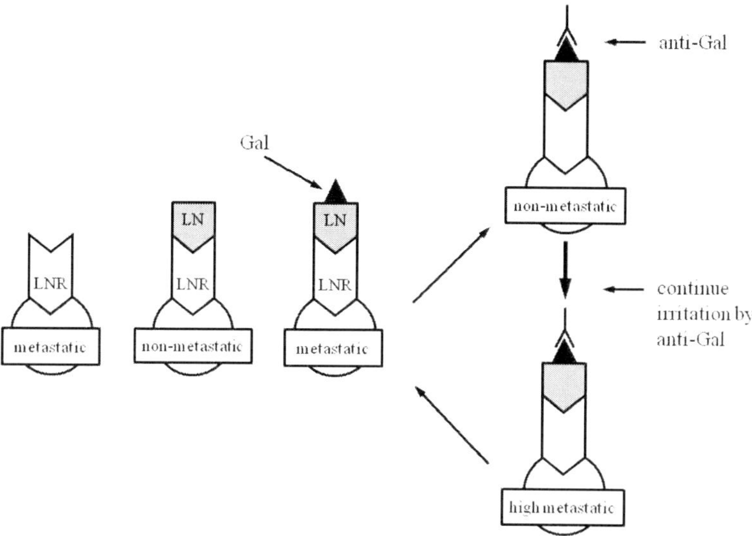

Figure 57. Hypothesis related to the relationship between cell surface laminin (LN) or LN containing α-Gal-containing oligosaccharide residues and lung metastatic potential. Gal: α-Gal residue. This hypothesis proposes that tumor cells without laminin receptors (LNRs) are not metastatic and that cells with empty LNRs are metastatic. Tumor cells with LNRs occupied by LN with or without α-Gal-containing oligosaccharide residues are metastatic and not metastatic, respectively. Tumor cells with the LN-Gal complex temporarily lose metastatic potential when incubated with anti-LN antibody or human blood group type A serum, but their metastatic potential is dramatically augmented when the cells are cultured with these substances for a long period. Because expression of α-Gal-containing oligosaccharide residues by 74FL cells decreased when they were cultured with human blood group type A serum, we believe that other unknown factors appear to modulate their metastatic potential [61].

However, when the various cell lines were cultured in medium supplemented with 10% human type A serum for more than ten days, the lung metastatic potential of 74AD and 74FL cells, which expressed the GS-I-B4-binding carbohydrate (recognizing terminal α-Gal residues) was dramatically increased; no such changes in metastatic potential were found with 74AD-f and 74FL-a cells, which rarely expressed the α-Gal-containing oligosaccharide residue (Table 10) [61]. Therefore, we postulate that anti-blood group type B antibody in blood group type A serum bound to cell surface LN-like molecules having oligosaccharides with terminal α-Gal residues and suppressed metastatic potential; however, treatment for a long period induced production of new factor(s) associated with enhancement of metastatic potential in a reversible fashion (Figure 57).

Two possible mechanisms for the biological activities of cell surface LN-like substances in tumor cell metastasis have been proposed [62,63]: 1) interaction between tumor cells and type IV collagen (CL-IV) substrates and 2) protection of tumor cells from natural killer cells and natural cytotoxic lymphocytes. The former possibility seems unlikely in our system because 74FL cells that express α-Gal-containing oligosaccharide residues on their surfaces rarely adhere to type IV collagen (CL-IV) substrates. The latter possibility should be investigated, however, because our previous study demonstrated that a high lung-colonizing potential of 74FL cells may be mediated by escape from natural host defense mechanisms [50]. Other studies have suggested that human natural anti-Gal antibodies act on the antitumor defense system, although the precise nature of the molecule(s) bearing α-Gal residues in tumor cells has yet to be determined [64,65].

Chapter VIII

CARBOHYDRATE EXPRESSION OF TUMOR CELLS AND ITS RELEVANCE TO METASTASIS AND PROGNOSIS

1. ANALYSIS OF HUMAN CANCERS

Our studies suggest that metastasis is intimately associated with the interaction of tumor cells and host tissues, especially with respect to cell surface adhesion molecules including carbohydrates. Therefore, we expanded our investigations to include extracellular matrix (ECM) proteins and carbohydrates as related to metastasis of human cancers. Our purpose at first was to determine, by using formalin-fixed and paraffin-embedded surgical specimens, whether expression of ECM proteins and/or carbohydrates of human tumor cells was associated with metastasis. We had clinical and pathological data available from more than 1,000 cases of breast, lung, gastric, colorectal, bile duct, and other cancers. The information included metastasis-related parameters such as lymphatic invasion (ly factor), venous invasion (v factor), metastasis, nerve invasion, and survival of patients followed up for about 15 years.

Preliminary examination of expression of FN, LN, CL-IV, and HSPG generated very limited insight, although we found a relationship between LN accumulation in cancer cell cytoplasm and lymph node metastasis in endometrial cancer [66]. In contrast, preliminary examination of carbohydrates led us to a new area of investigation because there were great differences among cancer cases in carbohydrate expression by cancer cells. Considerable attention was paid to abnormal carbohydrate expression in various kinds of human cancers [67]. Thus, we focused our studies on the relationship between carbohydrate expression by cancer cells in primary sites and metastatic potential [68-89]. The main reagents used to detect carbohydrates are listed in Table 11.

Table 11. Lectins and monoclonal antibodies used for carbohydrate detection

Lectins	Abbreviation	Main carbohydrate specificity
Griffonia Bandeirea simplicifolia isolectin B4	GS-I-B4	Galα1-3Gal
Artocarpus integrifolia	Jacalin	Galβ1-3GalNAc-Ser/Tre (T antigen)
Maclura pomifera	MPA	Melibiose
Helix pomatia	HPA	GalNAα1-3(Fuc1-2)Galβ1
Vicia villosa	VVA	GalNAc-O-Ser/Thr (Tn antigen)
Glycine max	SBA	Tn antigen
Dolichos biflorus	DBA	GalNAcα1-3(fuc1-2)Gal
Ricinus communis I	RCA-I	Galβ1-4GlcNAcβ1-
Ricinus communis II	RCA-II	Galβ1-4GlcNAcβ1-
Arachis hypogaea	PNA	Galβ1-3GalNAc-Ser/Thr (T antigen)
Erythrina cristagalli	ECA	Galβ1-4GlcNAc
Agaricus bisporus	ABA	Gal-GalNAc
Lotus tetragonolobus	Lotus	α-L-Fucose
Anguilla anguilla	AAA	α-L-Fucose
Ulex europaeus I	UEA-I	α1-2Fucose
Phaseolus vulgaris-L	PHA-L	GlcNAcβ1-6Manα1-6Man
Triticum vulgare	WGA	β-GlcNAc α-NeuAc
Canavalia ensiformis	ConA	α-Mannose
Lens culinaris	LCH	α-Mannose
MAbs		Main carbohydrate specificity
HB-T1		T antigen
HB-Tn1		Tn antigen
HB-STn1		NeuAcα2-6GalNAcα1-O-Ser/Thr (Sialyl-Tn antigen)
anti-blood group A	anti-A	Blood group substance A
anti-blood group B	anti-B	Blood group substance B
anti-blood group H	anti-H	Blood group substance H type 2
LEX-2		Lewis^{x} (Le^{x})
FH-6		sialyl dimeric Lewis$^{x\text{-}i}$ (SLe$^{x\text{-}i}$)
NS19-9		sialyl Lewis^{a} (SLe^{a})

Lectins were primarily purchased from EY Laboratory, San Mateo, CA.

2. Relationship of Carbohydrate Expression to Metastasis and Prognosis

Some of our results are presented in Table 12 and Figure 58. We confirmed that tumor cell carbohydrate expression in several types of cancer is significantly related to ly and v factors, metastasis, and prognosis, as many workers showed previously.

Table 12. Cancer cell carbohydrate expression as related to metastasis and prognosis of several human cancers

Type of primary cancer	Lymphatic vessel invasion (ly factor)	Blood vessel invasion (v factor)	Lymph node metastasis	Peritoneal metastasis	Liver metstasis	Prognosis	No. of cases [references]
Lung cancer							
Squamous cell carcinoma	ne	ne	HB-T1↑, HPA↑	ne	ne	HPA↑, VVA↑	100 cases [70]
Adenocarcinoma	PNA↑	-	PNA↑	ne	ne	-	164 cases [81]
Gastric cancer							
With submucosal invasion	ECA↓	UEA↓	RCA-I↓, WGA↓, ConA↓, HB-STn1↑	ne	ne	ne	118 cases [78]
With invasion into muscularis mucosa, serosa or exposed to abdominal wall	PHA-L↓, HB-T1↑, HB-Tn1↑, HB-STn1↑	HPA↓, AAA↓, Lotus↓, WGA↑, HB-T1↑, HB-Tn1↑, HB-STn1↑, FH-6↑	MPA↑, AAA↓, PHA-L↓, HB-STn1↑, FH-6↑	HPA↑, AAA↓, HB-STn1↑	ECA↓	HB-STn1↑, PHA-L↓	209 cases [74]
Colorectal cancer	MPA↑, PNA↑	DBA↑, LEX-2↑, FH-6↑	HPA↑	VVA↑	AAA↑, LEX-2↑, FH-6↑, NS19-9↑	FH-6↑, MPA↑	134 cases [79]

These studies were carried out with formalin-fixed and paraffin-embedded specimens without any pretreatment incubation. ↑ and ↓, indicate higher and lower values correlated with metastasis and prognosis, respectively; ne indicates not examined; – indicates no reagents that are related to metastasis and prognosis.

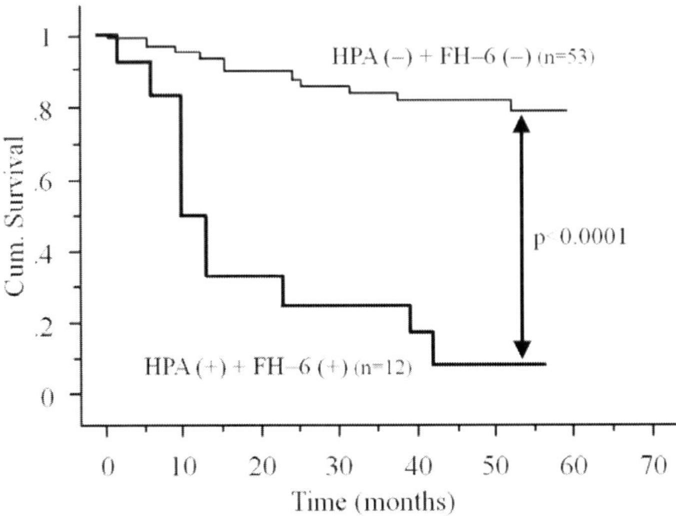

Figure 58. Additive effect of HPA and FH-6 staining. Cumulative survival of the HPA (–)/FH-6 (–) group, and HPA(+)/FH-6 (+) groups was markedly different [79].

For example, overexpression of HB-STn1-binding carbohydrate (STn antigen) in gastric cancer cells and FH-6 binding carbohydrate {sialyl dimeric Lewis^{x-i} (SLe^{x-i})} in colorectal cancer cells was related significantly to poor prognosis. Overexpression of the carbohydrates Le^{x}, SLe^{x-i}, and SLe^{a} in colorectal cancer cells was related to liver metastasis. Overexpression of HPA-binding carbohydrates in lung squamous cancer cells and colorectal cancer cells was related to lymph node metastases. These results were consistent with those of several previous reports [90-92].

It was interesting to find that low expression of *Phaseolus vulgaris*-L (PHA-L)-binding carbohydrate in gastric cancer cells was related to poor prognosis. It has been well documented that expression of PHA-L-binding carbohydrate by cancer cells is positively related to lung metastatic potential and/or poor prognosis not only in experimental murine tumors but also in several human cancers (colorectal cancer, breast cancer and malignant lymphoma), although some researchers have failed to confirm this finding [93-96]. The relationship between the expression of PHA-L-binding carbohydrate and metastasis or prognosis seems to differ in various cancers.

Our investigations also resulted in identification of several new reagents for predicting metastasis and/or prognosis, especially the lectins of GS-I-B4, MPA, AAA, and VVA. We previously described GS-I-B4 in detail. Here, we briefly describe MPA and AAA lectins. MPA binds specific galactose β1-3-*N*-

acetyl-D-galactosamine (Galβ1-3GalNAc) residues including Thomsen-Friedenreich (T) antigen, but it also binds T-like antigen [97]. AAA is one of the lectins that bind to blood group type H antigen (Fucα1-2Galβ1-3GlcNAc), but it also binds blood group type H-like antigen [98]. Because the staining pattern with these lectins and the staining with corresponding monoclonal antibodies (MAbs) (HB-T1 and anti-blood group H, respectively) were not the same, we believe that these lectins bind carbohydrate epitopes that are different from T and blood group type H antigens, respectively. This is also true of the carbohydrates *N*-acetyl-D-galactosamine (GalNAc, residues) that were recognized by VVA lectin and anti-Tn MAb. These results will be described in detail below.

3. Tumor Cell Carbohydrate Expression As a Determinant for the Route of Tumor Spread and Metastatic Pattern

Another interesting possibility arising from our studies is that certain kinds of carbohydrates in colorectal cancer cells in primary lesions may be related to the route of tumor cell spread and metastatic pattern (Table 12). MPA, HPA, VVA, and PNA are all Gal/GalNAc-specific lectins, thus it seems likely that the lymphatic spread (ly factor) of colorectal cancer cells is related to their expression of Gal/GalNAc residues. In contrast, venous spread (v factor) correlated with the carbohydrates recognized by DBA, LEX, FH-6, and NS19-9, which was related to liver metastasis (H factor). All the lectins and MAbs that showed correlations with v factor and H factor have in common the characteristic of binding to fucosylated carbohydrates. The finding that expression of Gal/GalNAc residues on colorectal cancer cells is one of the characteristics of cancer cells that spread into the lymphatic system is consistent with our knowledge about several cancers, such as breast, lung, and gastric cancer (Table 12). Although we do not know the exact biological function of the Gal/GalNAc residues expressed on cancer cells, in lymphatic metastasis, there are several possibilities. One is that these residues play a role in cancer cell traffic to the lymphatic system. Irimura et al. [99] has demonstrated that Gal/GalNAc-specific animal lectins are expressed on macrophages in lymph nodes and the peritoneal cavity. Another possibility is that Gal/GalNAc is associated with the invasion potential of cancer cells, probably mediated by adhesion of cancer cells to the ECM [100]. From one report, it seems likely that HPA-binding carbohydrates are associated with the immune response [101]. It is well known, however, that SLe^a and SLe^x antigens are, at least in part, ligands of the selectin family, especially E-selectin, which is expressed on activated endothelial cells in tiny blood vessels around colorectal cancer tissues and metastatic foci in the liver [102,103]. Therefore, it is reasonable to expect that SLe^a and SLe^x antigens expressed on colorectal cancer cells are utilized, in part, to form hematogenous liver metastases [104].

Overexpression of Gal/GalNAc on colorectal cancer cells may be caused by glycosyltransferase defects, as King et al. demonstrated [105]. In contrast, fucosyltransferase may contribute to increased expression of AAA-binding carbohydrates, Le^x, SLe^x, and SLe^a [106]. Although the precise mechanism of carbohydrates of tumor cells in tumor cell spread is not known, it is possible that lectins in the lymphatic system and selectins in the vascular system share routes of tumor cell spread and metastatic pattern via the carbohydrates expressed by tumor cells. One interesting study demonstrated positive correlation between Tn antigen expression and p53 protein expression by breast cancer cells and gastric cancer cells [39]. This result suggests that p53 protein may be related to the expression of immature mucin-type carbohydrate, but further study is needed to define the precise mechanism.

4. Application of Combination Analysis

As described above, the carbohydrates expressed by cancer cells have received much attention as molecules related to metastasis and prognosis. However, sometimes the relationship is not so strong as expected. There may be several reasons for this: (1) difficulty in estimation because of heterogeneous expression, (2) damage of glycoproteins during fixation and embedding, (3) dynamic changes in glycoproteins during tumor progression, and so on [92,107].

We think that a relationship between carbohydrate expression and metastasis or prognosis may exist, but metastasis-related pathological phenomena are too complex to be explained only as related to individual carbohydrates. For example, ly factor (tumor cells in lymphatic vessels) is a result of at least two different steps: tumor cell adhesion to the lymphatic wall and translocation of tumor cells into the vascular lumen. Each step apparently involves numerous molecular assemblies, and several kinds of tumor cell carbohydrates are used in each assembly. Combination analysis of tumor cell carbohydrate expression has been used to predict, with some precision, the lymph node metastasis of early gastric cancers as well as the prognosis of patients with colorectal cancer [78, 79]. To confirm the utility of using combination carbohydrate expression analysis, we examined the relationship between carbohydrate expression of cancer cells in primary lesions and lymph node metastasis of breast cancer, through analysis of the relationship between carbohydrate expression as recognized by two kinds of lectins and/or MAbs and lymph node metastasis status (Table 13). We found that 31 combinations of two lectins and/or MAbs correlate significantly with lymph node metastasis. Single lectins and MAbs, however, rarely correlate with lymph node metastasis [88]. These combinations form a completely interrelated linkage (or network) when all lectins and MAbs in the combinations are connected with one another (Figure 59). The network included linkages among anti-Tn, VVA, anti-H, AAA, and anti-Le^x in the center; VVA occupied the central core, which may be due to VVAs being the only reagent among them significantly related to lymphatic invasion (ly factor).

Table 13. Statistical assessment of synergistic and antagonistic relationships for lymph node metastasis and two kinds of lectins or monoclonal antibodies

Staining status by two kinds of lectins or MAbs [a]		No. of cases [b]		Node-positive (%)
A	B	n(–)	n(+)	
–	–	a	b	① [b/a + b]×100
+	–	c	d	② [d/c + d]×100
–	+	e	f	③ [f/ e + f]×100
+	+	g	h	④ [h/g + h]×100

[a]: + and – indicate positive and negative staining by lectins or MAbs. [b]: n(–) and n(+) mean lymph node metastasis-negative and-positive cases, respectively. Positive or negative staining was defined as >50% or≦50% of stained cells for lectins and >10% or ≦10% of stained cells for MAbs, respectively. There are four possible: {–, –}, {+, –}, {–, +}, and {+, +}, by combination of A and B reagents (i.e., lectin or MAb). When there was a statistically significant difference for lymph node metastasis-positive percentages between ④ and ①, the pair of reagents was considered to have a synergistic relationship. The pair of reagents was considered to have an antagonistic relationship when there was a statistically significant difference between ② and ③. Statistical analysis of differences between groups was performed by the χ^2 test, with the continuity correction of Yates. A p value <0.05 was considered significant.

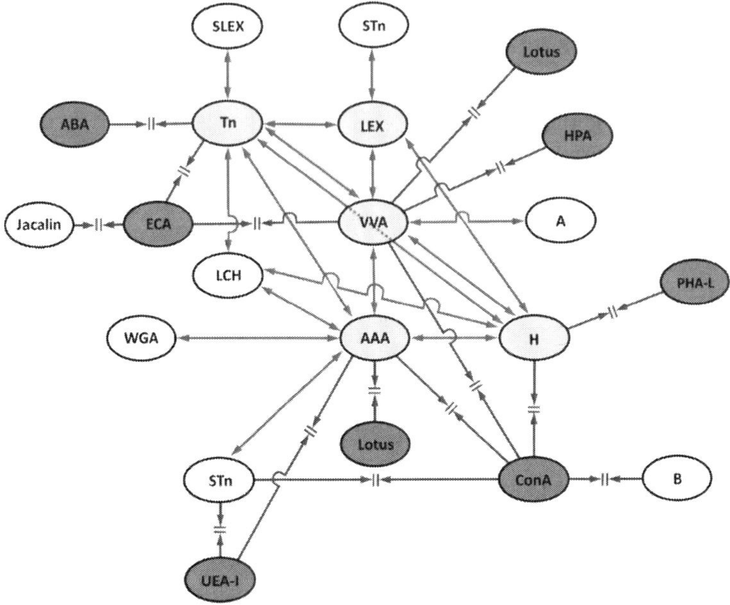

Figure 59. Lymph node metastasis-related carbohydrate network for breast cancer. Combination analysis revealed that 31 combinations had a significant correlation with lymph node metastasis. These combinations formed a completely closed linkage (or network) when lectins and MAbs were connected by lines indicating a significant ($p < 0.05$) relationship between them. The network included linkage among HB-Tn1, VVA, anti-H, AAA, and LEX-2 in the center, with VVA occupying the central core. VVA was the reagent whose staining was related to the ly factor, which suggests that lymph node metastasis occurs when VVA-reactive carbohydrate(s) develop [88].

5. Tn Antigen As Molecular Determinant(s) of ly Factor

5.1. Invasive Ductal Carcinoma of Breast

We continue to study the carbohydrate epitope and molecules having VVA-binding carbohydrates in human breast cancer. Results have shown that VVA recognizes the GalNAc residue of glycoprotein in cancer cells, which resembles Tn antigen (GalNAcα1-O-Ser/Thr), as indicated by other workers [108]; but the carbohydrate recognized by VVA is not identical to it. VVA bound either GalNAcα-1-O-PAP-HSA or GalNAcβ-1-O-PAP-HSA. Our study also demonstrated that under denaturing and reducing conditions, the major

VVA- binding proteins had molecular sizes of >200 kDa, ~75 kDa, ~50 kDa, ~33 kDa., and ~26 kDa. The >200 kDa, ~75 kDa, ~50 kDa and ~26 kDa proteins were identified as MUC1 mucin, serotransferrin, IgG heavy chain, and IgG light chain, respectively. Expression of the ~33 kDa protein was most relevant to lymph node metastasis; this protein may be MUC1 (Figure 60). More recently, we discovered that liver metastasis of breast cancer is related to expression of proteins with VVA-binding carbohydrates. Metastatic cancer cells in the liver and the corresponding primary breast cancer cells frequently stained with VVA (52.6%±28.9, N=10, and 44.5%±31.1, N=10, respectively), whereas primary breast cancer cells stained infrequently with VVA (19.4%±16.5, N=7), when no metastasis in the liver was found at autopsy. Liver tissues with metastasis were harvested from two autopsy cases, and VVA-binding proteins were examined by sodium dodecyl sulphate-polyacrylamide gel electrophoresis (SDS-PAGE) followed by Western blotting . VVA binding was mainly found at ~50, ~65, 120, and >450 kDa in one case, and at ~10, ~25, 30, ~33, ~44, and ~50 in the other case. The ~10, ~25, 30, ~50, and >450 kDa molecules are thought to be MUC1 on the basis of the reactivity of VU-3C6 mouse anti-MUC1 monoclonal antibody; the ~33, 44, and ~120 kDa proteins remain to be identified. This result indicates that VVA-binding carbohydrates are carried on atypical MUC1.

Although the exact epitope structures of VVA-binding carbohydrate(s) and the carrier protein(s) remain to be studied, we believe that VVA-binding carbohydrates on MUC1 of cancer cells are an important molecular drug target in aggressive breast cancer. It is likely that VVA-binding carbohydrates are an important molecular target in other cancers as well because VVA-binding carbohydrate expression is related to the malignant phenotype of various human cancers including lung cancer, uterine cervical cancer, colon cancer, pancreatic cancer, urinary bladder cancer, and malignant lymphoma.

5.2. Rat Ascites Hepatoma AH109A Cells

In addition to human cancers, we are investigating aberrant MUC1 bearing Tn antigen of rat ascites hepatoma AH109A cells (poorly differentiated hepatocellular carcinoma) with strong lymphatic metastasis propensity [87]. These cells metastasized to lymph nodes two to three weeks after subcutaneous (sc) inoculation of abdominal wall when intercellular adhesion molecule 1 (ICAM-1) appeared in vascular endothelial cells around the tumor. AH109A cells, mainly in their cytoplasm, contained a considerable amount of substances reactive to VVA and anti-MUC1 antibody raised against to amino acids 961-1255 mapping at the C-terminus of MUC1 of human antigen. SDS-PAGE analyses followed by Western blotting demonstrated that primary tumor cells and metastatic tumor cells possessed mainly MUC1 proteins of 30~40 kDa, as purified via affinity chromatography with VVA column and peanut lectin column (Figure 61).

VVA-reactivity of 30-40 kDa proteins of the primary tumor cells was completely absorbed after pre-incubation with 1 mM of Tn antigen (*N*-acetylgalactosamine-*O*-Ser/Thr). Antibodies raised against N-terminal and C-terminal regions did not react with these MUC1 proteins of 30~40 kDa bearing Tn antigen.

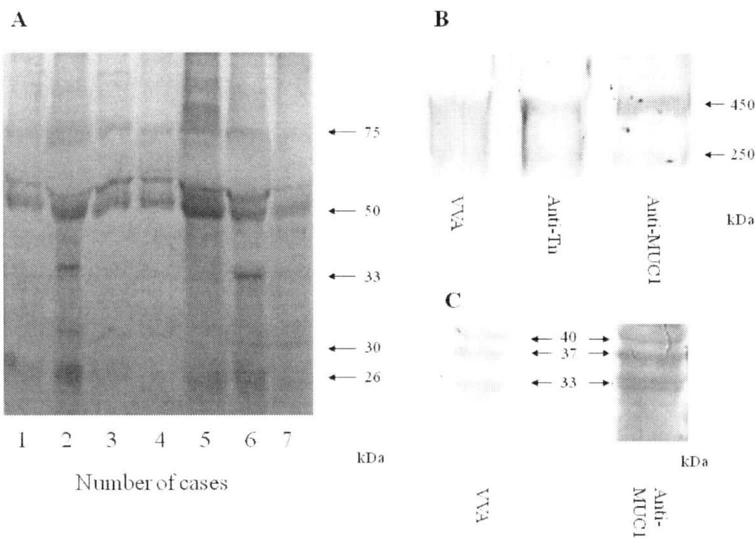

Figure 60. A: Expression of VVA-binding proteins in human breast cancer demonstrated by Western blotting. Results for proteins of relatively low molecular size from seven cases of primary cancer are shown. The protein with a molecular size of ~33 kDa was the most relevant to lymph node metastasis. B: VVA-, HB-Tn1, and VU-3C6-positive molecules with molecular sizes greater than 200 kDa. One case served as the source of samples used in all staining evaluations. VVA-positive bands sometimes appeared smeared; therefore, the precise molecular size was difficult to estimate. Staining-positive bands from HB-Tn1 (anti-Tn) and VU-3C6 (anti-MUC1) appeared to be located at 250 and 450 kDa, respectively. C: VU-3C6-positive molecules with molecular sizes of ~33, ~37, and ~40 kDa, but not ~30 kDa, were found in this breast cancer case [85].

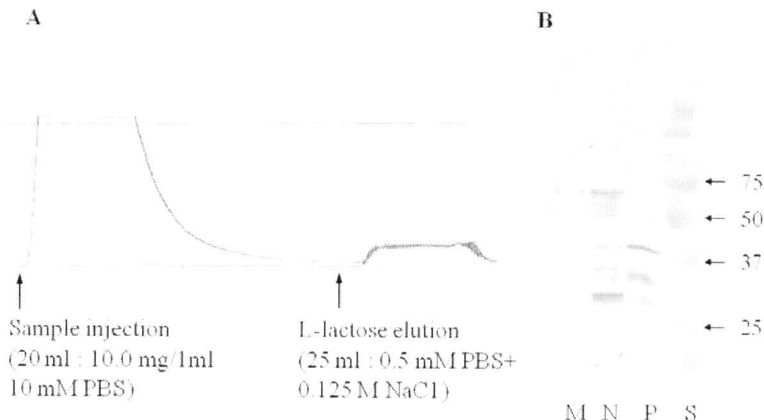

Figure 61. MUC1 of rat ascites hepatoma AH109A tumors purified by PNA affinity chromatography. A: PNA affinity chromatography. B: Western blotting profiles of P (primary sc tumor), N (lymph node metastasis), and M (submaxillary mucin for control) in denaturing and reducing conditions. Anti-MUC1 antibody H-295-positive bands were detected using alkaline phosphatase. S, standard molecules [87].

We conclude that rat ascites hepatoma AH109 cells express an aberrant type of MUC1 proteins of 30~40 kDa bearing VVA-reactive carbohydrate(s) (Tn antigen). These aberrant MUC1 proteins bearing Tn antigen appear to be derived from extracellular sequence of C-terminal subunit or transmembrane domain of MUC1, suggesting that these aberrant MUC1 proteins are SEA module of MUC1. So, aberrant MUC1 proteins may participate in lymphatic metastasis via release and binding of tumor cells, but we do not know the role of Tn antigen born by MUC1, which appear in primary tumor cells.

References

[1] Yonemura, Y; Oyama, S; Sugiyama, K; Sawa, T; Shima, Y; Kamata, T; Hashimoto, T; Miwa, K; Miyazaki, I. Human chorionic gonadotropin in gastric carcinoma. A useful marker for bone metastasis. *Int. Surg.*, 1989, 74, 84-87.

[2] Morife, R; Lorigan, P; MacNeil, S. Gender and survival in malignant tumours. *Cancer Treat. Rev.*, 2001, 27, 201-209.

[3] Enzinger, FM; Weiss, SW. General consideration. In: Enzinger FM, Weiss SW, editors. *Soft tissue tumors* ,Fifth ed., St Loius: Mosby; 2008; 1-14.

[4] Nessar, H. Carcinoma with micropapillary morphology: clinical significance and current concepts. *Adv. Anat. Pathol.*, 2004, 11, 297-303.

[5] Weidner, N; Semple, JP; Welch, WR; Folkman, J. Tumor angiogenesis and metastasis-correlation in invasive breast carcinoma. *N. Engl. J. Med.*, 1991, 324, 1-8.

[6] Hasebe, T; Imoto, S; Sasaki, S; Mukai, K. A proposal for a new histological classification scheme for predicting short-term tumor recurrence and death in patients with invasive ductal carcinoma of the breast. *Jpn. J. Cancer Res.*, 1998, 89, 1358-1373.

[7] Partin, AW; Schoeniger, JS; Mohler, JL; Coffey, DS. Fourier analysis of cell motility: correlation of motility with metastatic potential. *Proc. Natl. Acad. Sci. USA*, 1989, 86, 1254-1258.

[8] Taniguchi, S; Kawano, T; Kakunaga, T; Baba, T. Differences in expression of a variant actin between low and high metastatic B16 melanoma. *J. Biol. Chem.*, 1986, 261, 6100-6106.

[9] Raz, A; Ben-Ze'ev, A. Modulation of the metastatic capability in B16 melanoma by cell shape. *Science*, 1983, 221, 1307-1310.

[10] Kawaguchi, T; Watanabe, K; Sugino, T; Saito, A; Igarashi, S; Ono, T; Nakamura, K; Yokoya, S; Ozawa, M; Muramatsu, T. Establishment and characterization of metastatic ascites hepatoma variants with different adhesive properties to substrate in vitro. In: Ikawa Y, Wada A, editors. *Recent Progress of Life Science Technology in Japan*. Tokyo: Academic Press; 1989; 267-279.

[11] Kawaguchi, T; Igarashi, S; Wakabayashi, H; Yokoya, S; Fukui, K. Substrate adhesiveness and experimental metastatic potential of rat ascites hepatoma AH7974-derived variant sublines. *Clin. Exp. Metastasis*, 1992, 10, 225-238.

[12] Nomura, Y; Tashiro, H; Hisamatsu, K. In vitro clonogenic growth and metastatic potential of human operable breast cancer. *Cancer Res.*, 1989, 49, 5288-5293.

[13] Cohen, S. Isolation of a mouse submaxillary gland protein accelerating incisor eruption and eyelid opening in the new-born animal. *J. Biol. Chem.*, 1962, 237, 1555-1562.

[14] Khazaie, K; Schirrmacher, V; Lichtner, RB. EGF receptor in neoplasia and metastasis. *Cancer Metastasis Rev.*, 1993, 12, 255-274.

[15] Kusukawa, J; Harada, H; Shima, I; Sasaguri, Y; Kameyama, T; Morimatsu, M. The significance of epidermal growth factor receptor and matrix metalloproteinase-3 in squamous cell carcinoma of the oral cavity. *Eur. J. Cancer B. Oral Oncol.*, 1996, 32B, 217-221.

[16] Welch, DR; Fabra, A; Nakajima, M. Transforming growth factor β stimulates mammary adenocarcinoma cell invasion and metastatic potential. *Proc. Natl. Acad. Sci. USA*, 1990, 87, 7678-7682.
[17] Fidler, IJ; Ellis, LM. The implications of angiogenesis for the biology and therapy of cancer metastasis. *Cell*, 1994, 79, 185-188.
[18] Ueoka, Y; Kato, K; Kuriaki, Y; Horiuchi, S; Terao, Y; Nishida, J; Ueno, H; Wake, N. Hepatocyte growth factor modulates motility and invasiveness of ovarian carcinomas via Ras-mediated pathway. *Br. J. Cancer*, 2000, 82, 891-899.
[19] Nabi, IR; Watanabe, H; Raz, A. Autocrine motility factor and its receptor: role in cell locomotion and metastasis. *Cancer Metastasis Rev.*, 1992, 11, 5-20.
[20] Watanabe, H; Takehana, K; Date, M; Shinozaki, T; Raz, A. Tumor cell autocrine motility factor is the neuroleukin/phosphohexose isomerase polypeptide. *Cancer Res.*, 1996, 56, 2960-2963.
[21] Kleer, CG; van Golen, KL; Zhang, Y; Wu, ZF; Rubin, MA; Merajver, SD. Characterization of RhoC expression in benign and malignant breast disease: a potential new marker for small breast carcinomas with metastatic ability. *Am. J. Pathol.*, 2002, 160, 579-584.
[22] Yoshizaki, N; Mogi, Y; Muramatsu, H; Koike, K; Kogawa, K; Niitsu, Y. Suppressive effect of recombinant human Cu, Zn-superoxide dismutase on lung metastasis of murine tumor cells. *Int. J. Cancer*, 1994, 57, 287-292.
[23] Liotta, LA; Tryggvason, K; Garbisa, S; Hart, I; Foltz, CM; Shafie, S. Metastatic potential correlates with enzymatic degradation of basement membrane collagen. *Nature*, 1980, 284, 67-68.
[24] Nakajima, M; Irimura, T; Di Ferrante, D; Di Ferrante, N; Nicolson, GL. Heparan sulfate degradation: relation to tumor invasive and metastatic properties of mouse B16 melanoma sublines. *Science*, 1983, 220, 611-613.
[25] Tanaka, K; Kohga, S; Kinjyo, M; Kodama, Y. Tumor metastasis and thrombosis, with special reference to thromboplastic and fibrinolytic activities of tumor cells. *Gann Monogr. Cancer Res.*, 1977, 20, 97-119.
[26] Hejna, M; Raderer, M; Zielinski, CC. Inhibition of metastases by anticoagulants. *J. Natl. Cancer Inst.*, 1999, 91, 22-36.
[27] Frost, P; Kerbel, RS. Immunology of metastasis. Can the immune response cope with disseminated tumor? *Cancer Metastasis Rev.*, 1983, 2, 239-256.
[28] Levy, EM; Roberti, MP; Mordoh, J. Natural killer cells in human cancer:

from biological functions to clinical applications. *J. Biomed. Biotechnol.*, 2011, Epub, ahead of print.

[29] Mansfield, AS; Heikkila, P; von Smitten, K; Vakkila, J; Leidenius, M. Metastasis to sentinel lymph nodes in breast cancer is associated with maturation arrest of dendritic cells and poor co-localization of dendritic cells and $CD8^+$ T cells. *Virchows Arch.*, 2011, 459, 391-398.

[30] Tsuda, T; Tahara, E; Kajiyama, G; Sakamoto, H; Terada, M; Sugimura, T. High incidence of coamplification of hst-1 and int-2 genes in human esophageal carcinomas. *Cancer Res.*, 1989, 49, 5505-5508.

[31] Shinozaki, H; Ozawa, S; Ando, N; Tsuruta, H; Terada, M; Ueda, M; Kitajima, M. Cyclin D1 amplification as a new predictive classification for squamous cell carcinoma of the esophagus, adding gene information. *Clin. Cancer Res.*, 1996, 2, 1155-1161.

[32] Hattori, Y; Itoh, H; Uchino, S; Hosokawa, K; Ochiai, A; Ino, Y; Ishii, H; Sakamoto, H; Yamaguchi, N; Yanagihara, K; Hirohashi, S; Sugimura, T; Terada, M. Immunohistochemical detection of K-sam protein in stomach cancer. *Clin. Cancer Res.*, 1996, 2, 1373-1381.

[33] Vogelstein, B; Fearon, ER; Hamilton, SR; Kern, SE; Preisinger, AC; Leppert, M; Nakamura, Y; White, R; Smits, AM; Bos, JL. Genetic alterations during colorectal-tumor development. *N. Engl. J. Med.*, 1988, 319, 525-532.

[34] Almoguera, C; Shibata, D; Forrester, K; Martin, J; Arnheim, N; Perucho, M. Most human carcinomas of the exocrine pancreas contain mutant c-K-ras genes. *Cell*, 1988, 53, 549-554.

[35] Brodeur, GM; Seeger, RC; Schwab, M; Varmus, HE; Bishop, JM. Amplification of N-myc in untreated human neuroblastomas correlates with advanced disease stage. *Science*, 1984, 224, 1121-1124.

[36] Taniguchi, S; Nishimura, Y; Takahashi, T; Baba, T; Kato, K. Augmented excretion of procathepsin L of a fos-transferred highly metastatic rat cell line. *Biochem. Biophys. Res. Commun.*, 1990, 168, 520-526.

[37] Koyama, S; Terashima, S; Takano, Y; Ohori, T; Inoue, H; Motoki, R; Kawaguchi, T. P53 protein expression of carcinoma cells associated with metastasis and prognosis in gastric carcinomas: a clinicopathological study. *Fukushima Igaku Zasshi*, 1997, 47, 131-142. (in Japanese).

[38] Suzuki, H; Kawaguchi, T; Hasegawa, T; Yonechi, A; Ohsugi, J; Higuchi, M; Yamada, F; Shio, Y; Fujiu, K; Kanno, R; Ohishi, A; Gotoh, M. Prognostic impact of p53 protein overexpression in patients with node-negative lung adenocarcinoma. *Cancer Lett.*, 2006, 237, 242-247.

[39] Kawaguchi, T; Takano, Y; Ohori, T; Ito, F; Koyama, S; Kanno, T. Carbohydrate expression of tumor cells in progression of gastric cancer from early to advanced stage. *Stomach Intestine*, 1997, 32, 797-808. (in Japanese).

[40] Malik, FA; Sanders, AJ; Jiang, WG. KAI-1/CD82, the molecule and clinical implication in cancer and cancer metastasis. *Histol. Histopathol.*, 2009, 24, 519-530.

[41] Mihic-Probst, D; Mnich, CD; Oberholzer, PA; Seifert, B; Sasse, B; Moch, H; Dummer, R. p16 expression in primary malignant melanoma is associated with prognosis and lymph node status. *Int. J. Cancer*, 2006, 118, 2262-2268.

[42] Steeg, PS; Bevilacqua, G; Kopper, L; Thorgeirsson, UP; Talmadge, JE; Liotta, LA; Sobel, ME. Evidence for a novel gene associated with low tumor metastatic potential. *J. Natl. Cancer Inst.*, 1988, 80, 200-204.

[43] Kimura, N; Shimada, N; Nomura, K; Watanabe, K. Isolation and characterization of a cDNA clone encoding rat nucleoside diphosphate kinase. *J. Biol. Chem.*, 1990, 265, 15744-15749.

[44] Keirseblick, A; Bonné, S; Bruyneel, E; Vermassen, P; Lukanidin, E; Mareel, M; van Roy, F. E-cadherin and metastasin (mts-1/S100A4) expression levels are inversely regulated in two tumor cell families. *Cancer Res.*, 1998, 58, 4587-4591.

[45] Denhardt, DT. Oncogene-initiated aberrant signaling engenders the metastatic phenotype: synergistic transcription factor interactions are targets for cancer therapy. *Crit. Rev. Oncog.*, 1996, 7, 261-291.

[46] Liotta, LA. Tumor invasion and metastases--role of the extracellular matrix: Rhoads Memorial Award lecture. *Cancer Res.*, 1986, 46, 1-7.

[47] Nicolson, GL. Organ specificity of tumor metastasis: role of preferential adhesion, invasion and growth of malignant cells at specific secondary sites. *Cancer Metastasis Rev.*, 1988, 7, 143-188.

[48] Klein, E. Gradual transformation of solid into ascites tumors. Evidence favoring the mutation-selection theory. *Exp. Cell Res.*, 1955, 8, 188-212.

[49] Yoshida, T. Contributions of the ascites hepatoma to the concept of malignancy of cancer. *Ann. N. Y. Acad. Sci.*, 1956, 63, 852-881.

[50] Kawaguchi, T; Ono, T; Wakabayashi, H; Igarashi, S. Cell surface laminin-like substances and laminin-related carbohydrates of rat ascites hepatoma AH7974 and its variants with different lung-colonizing potential. *Clin. and Exp. Metastasis*, 1994, 12, 203-212.

[51] Ono, T. Establishment and characterization of adherent and nonadherent tumor cell lines originated from rat ascites hepatoma AH7974 in serum-

free medium: their producibility of and adhesiveness to ECM protein and metastatic potency. *Fukushima Igaku Zasshi*, 1989, 39, 333-350. (in Japanese).

[52] Murray, JC; Liotta, L; Rennard, SI; Martin, GR. Adhesion characteristics of murine metastatic and nonmetastatic tumor cells in vitro. *Cancer Res.*, 1980, 40, 347-351.

[53] Bal de Kier Joffé, E; Puricelli, L; de Lustig, ES. Modified adhesion behavior after in vitro passage of two related murine mammary adenocarcinomas with different metastasizing ability. *Invasion Metastasis*, 1986, 6, 302-312.

[54] Terranova, VP; Liotta, LA; Russo, RG; Martin, GR. Role of laminin in the attachment and metastasis of murine tumor cells. *Cancer Res.*, 1982, 42, 2265-2269.

[55] Kimura, A; Kawaguchi, T; Ono, T; Sakuma, A; Yokoya, S; Kochi, H; Nakamura, K. Cell-surface heparan sulfate and adhesive property of sublines of rat ascites hepatoma AH7974. *J. Cell Sci.*, 1988, 90, 683-689.

[56] Sanderson, RD. Heparan sulfate proteoglycans in invasion and metastasis. *Semin. Cell Dev. Biol.*, 2001, 12, 89-98.

[57] Ozawa, M; Sato, M; Muramatsu, H; Hamada, H; Muramatsu, T. A membrane glycoprotein involved in teratocarcinoma cell adhesion to substratum. *Exp. Cell Res.*, 1985, 158, 127-143.

[58] Rieber, M; Castillo, MA; Rieber, MS; Irwin, JC; Urbina, C. Decrease in tumor cell attachment and in a 140-kDa fibronectin receptor correlate with greater expression of multiple 34-kDa surface proteins and cytoplasmic 54-kDa components. *Int. J. Cancer*, 1988, 41, 96-100.

[59] Blumenstock, FA; Saba, TM; Weber, P; Laffin, R. Biochemical and immunological characterization of human opsonic alpha 2SB glycoprotein: its identify with cold-insoluble globulin. *J. Biol. Chem.*, 1978, 253, 4287-4291.

[60] Varani, J; Lovett, EJ III; Wicha, M; Malinoff, H; McCoy, JP. Cell surface α-D-galactopyranol end groups: use as markers in the isolation of murine tumor cell lines with different cancer causing potential. *J. Natl. Cancer Inst.*, 1983, 71, 1281-1287.

[61] Kawaguchi, T; Kanno, M; Kimijima, I; Abe, R. Carbohydrate expression of tumor cells and prognosis of breast cancer-analysis on human cancer and experimental certification on mechanism. *Basic Invest. Breast Carcinoma*, 1997, 6, 41-47. (in Japanese).

[62] Grimstad, IA; Varani, J; McCoy, JP. Jr. Contribution of α-D-galactopyranoside end groups to attachment of highly and low

metastatic murine fibrosarcoma cells to various substrates. *Exp. Cell Res.*, 1984, 155, 345-358.
[63] Hiserodt, JC; Laybourn, KA; Varani, J. Laminin inhibits the recognition of tumor target cells by murine natural killer (NK) and natural cytotoxic (NC) lymphocytes. *Am. J. Pathol.*, 1985, 121, 148-155.
[64] Castronovo, V; Colin, C; Claysmith, AP; Chen, PH; Lifrange, E; Lambotte, R; Krutzsch, H; Liotta, LA; Sobel, ME. Immunodetection of the metastasis-associated laminin receptor in human breast cancer cells obtained by fine-needle aspiration biopsy. *Am. J. Pathol.*, 1990, 137, 1373-1381.
[65] Galili, U; Macher, BA. Interaction between anti-Gal and human tumor cells: a natural defense mechanism? *J. Natl. Cancer Inst.*, 1989, 81, 178-179.
[66] Ooishi, M; Kawaguchi, T; Hoshi, K; Morimura, Y; Sato, A; Suzuki, T. Immunohistochemical demonstration of laminin in endometrial cancer of uterus in relation to its invasion and metastasis. *Acta Obstet. Gynaecol. Jpn.*, 1995, 47, 955-956.
[67] Hakomori, S. Aberrant glycosylation in tumors and tumor-associated tumor antigens. *Adv. Cancer Res.*, 1989, 52, 257-331.
[68] Kawaguchi, T; Kanno, M; Kimijima, I; Abe, R. Lymph node metastasis-related carbohydrate network of tumor cells in primary breast cancer-complement. *Basic Invest. Breast Carcinoma*, 1996, 5, 33-36. (in Japanese).
[69] Terashima, S; Takano, Y; Ohori, T; Kanno, T; Kimura, T; Motoki, R; Kawaguchi, T. Soybean agglutinin binding as a useful prognostic indicator in stomach cancer. *Surg. Today*, 1997, 27, 293-297.
[70] Fujiu, K; Kawaguchi, T; Suzuki, H; Kushida, M; Kanno, R; Oishi, A; Inoue, H; Motoki, R. Expression of mucin type core carbohydrates in squamous cell carcinoma of the lung and its relationship to metastasis and outcome. *Lung Cancer*, 1997, 37, 301-311. (in Japanese).
[71] Kawaguchi, T. Adhesion molecules and carbohydrates in cancer metastasis. *Jpn. J. Clin. Pathol.*, 1996, 44, 1138-1146.
[72] Kawaguchi, T; Kanno, M; Kimijima, I; Abe, R. Lymph node metastasis-related carbohydrate network of tumor cells in primary breast cancer-complement. *Basic Invest. Breast Carcinoma*, 1998, 7, 59-63. (in Japanese).
[73] Terashima, S; Takano, Y; Ohori, T; Kanno, T; Kimura, T; Motoki, R; Kawaguchi, T. Sialyl-Tn antigen as a useful predictor of poor prognosis in patients with advanced stomach cancer. *Surg. Today*, 1998, 28, 682-

686.
[74] Ohori, T; Kawaguchi, T. Carbohydrate expression of carcinoma cells associated with metastasis and prognosis in advanced gastric carcinomas: a clinocopathological study. *Fukushima Igaku Zasshi*, 1998, 48, 25-36. (in Japanese).
[75] Tsuchiya, A; Kanno, M; Kawaguchi, T; Endo, Y; Zhang, GJ; Ohtake, T; Kimijima, I. Prognostic relevance of Tn expression in breast cancer. *Breast Cancer*, 1999, 6, 175-180.
[76] Suzuki, O; Nozawa, Y; Kawaguchi, T; Abe, M. Phaseolus vulgaris leukoagglutinating lectin-binding reactivity in human diffuse large B-cell lymphoma and its relevance to the patient's clinical outcome: Lectin histochemistry and lectin blot analysis. *Pathol. Int.*, 1999, 49, 874-880.
[77] Kawaguchi, T; Kanno, M; Kimijima, I; Takazawa, H; Imai, S; Hilgers, J. Is MUC1 a carrier protein of Tn antigen? Studies on molecules and clinicopathological parameters. *Basic Invest. Breast Carcinoma*, 1999, 8, 62-66. (in Japanese).
[78] Takano, Y; Teranishi, Y; Terashima, S; Motoki, R; Kawaguchi, T. Lymph node metastasis-related carbohydrates epitopes of gastric cancer with submucosal invasion. *Surg. Today*, 2000, 30, 1073-1082.
[79] Konno, A; Hoshino, Y; Terashima, S; Motoki, R; Kawaguchi, T. Carbohydrate expression profile of colorectal tumor cells is relevant to metastatic pattern and prognosis. *Clin. Exp. Metastasis*, 2002, 19, 61-70.
[80] Suzuki, O; Nozawa, Y; Kawaguchi, T; Abe, M. UDP-GlcNAc2-epimerase regulates cell surface sialylation and cell adhesion to extracellular matrix in Burkitt's lymphoma. *Int. J. Oncol.*, 2002, 20, 1005-1011.
[81] Suzuki, H; Kawaguchi, T; Higuchi, M; Shio, Y; Fujiu, K; Kanno, R; Ohishi, A; Motoki, R; Gotoh, M. Expression of peanut agglutinin-binding carbohydrates correlates with nodal involvement in human lung adenocarcinoma. *Cancer Lett.*, 2002, 187, 215-221.
[82] Suzuki, O; Nozawa, Y; Kawaguchi, T; Abe, M. Alpha-2,6-sialylation of L-PHA reactive oligosaccharides and expression of N-acetyl-glucosaminyltransferase V in human diffuse large B cell lymphoma. *Oncol. Rep.*, 2003, 10, 1759-1764.
[83] Kawaguchi, T. Cancer metastasis: characterization and identification of the behavior of metastatic tumor cells and the cell adhesion molecules, including carbohydrates. *Current Drug Targets Cardiovasc. Hematol. Dis.*, 2005, 5, 39-64.
[84] Kawaguchi, T; Takazawa, H; Imai, S; Morimoto, J; Watanabe, T. Lack

of polymorphism in MUC1 tandem repeats in cancer cells is related to breast cancer progression in Japanese woman. *Breast Cancer Res. Treat.*, 2005, 92, 223-230.

[85] Kawaguchi, T; Takazawa, H; Imai, S; Morimoto, J; Watanabe, T; Kanno, M; Igarashi, S. Expression of Vicia villosa agglutinin (VVA)-binding glycoprotein on primary breast cancer cells in relation to lymphatic metastasis: is atypical MUC1 bearing Tn antigen a receptor of VVA? *Breast Cancer Res. Treat.*, 2006, 98, 31-43.

[86] Shio, Y; Suzuki, H; Kawaguchi, T; Ohsugi, J; Higuchi, M; Fujiu, K; Kanno, R; Ohishi, A; Gotoh, M. Carbohydrate status detecting by PNA is changeable through cancer prognosis from primary to metastatic nodal site: a possible prognostic factor in patient with node-positive lung adenocarcinoma. *Lung cancer*, 2007, 57, 187-192.

[87] Kawaguchi, T; Imai, S; Haga, S; Morimoto, J; Honda, T. Demonstration and partial identification of aberrant Muc1 bearing Tn antigen in rat ascites hepatoma AH109A cells with strong lymph node metastasis propensity. In: Watanabe A, editor. *Cancer Metastasis Research*. New York: Nova Science Publishers; 2008; 147-163.

[88] Kawaguchi, T; Kanno, M; Takazawa, H; Imai, S; Morimoto, J; Haga, S; Honda, T. Lymphatic spreading propensity and aberrant MUC1 bearing TN/TN-like carbohydrate of aggressive breast cancer cells. In: DeFrina RH, editor. *Aggressive Breast Cancer*. New York: Nova Science Publishers; 2009; 199-228.

[89] Kawaguchi, T; Kanno, M; Asahi, S; Honda, T. Relationship between carbohydrate expression profiles of cancer cells and prognosis of breast cancer patients. In: DeFrina RH, editor. *Aggressive Breast Cancer*. New York: Nova Science Publishers; 2009; 231-235.

[90] Springer, GF. T and Tn, general carcinoma autoantigens. *Science*, 1984, 224, 1198-1206.

[91] Dabelsteen, E. Cell surface carbohydrates as prognostic markers in human carcinomas. *J. Pathol.*, 1996, 179, 358-369.

[92] Brooks, SA. The involvement of Helix pomatia lectin (HPA) binding N-acetylgalactosamine glycans in cancer progression. *Histol. Histopathol.*, 2000, 15, 143-158.

[93] Dennis, JW; Laferté, S; Waghorne, C; Breitman, ML; Kerbel, RS. β1-6 branching of Asn-linked oligosaccharides is directly associated with metastasis. *Science*, 1987, 236, 582-585.

[94] Seelentag, WK; Li, WP; Schmitz, SF; Metzger, U; Aeberhard, P; Heitz, PU; Roth, J. Prognostic value of β1,6-branched oligosaccharides in

human colorectal carcinoma. *Cancer Res.*, 1998, 58, 5559-5564.

[95] Fernandes, B; Sagman, U; Auger, M; Demetrio, M; Dennis, JW. β1-6 branched oligosaccharides as a marker of tumor progression in human breast and colon neoplasia. *Cancer Res.*, 1991, 51, 718-723.

[96] Chammas, R; Cella, N; Marques, LA; Brentani, RR; Hynes, NE; Franco, EL. Correspondence re: B. Fernandes et al., β1-6 branched oligosaccharides as a marker of tumor progression in human breast and colon neoplasia. Cancer Res., 51: 718-723, 1991. *Cancer Res.*, 54, 1994, 306-308.

[97] Macartney, JC. Lectin histochemistry of galactose and N-acetyl-galactosamine glycoproteins in normal gastric mucosa and gastric cancer and the relationship with ABO secretor status. *J. Pathol.*, 1986, 150, 135-144.

[98] Hammarström, S; Murphy, LA; Goldstein, IJ; Etzler, ME. Carbohydrate binding specificity of four N-acetyl-D-galactosamine-"specific" lectins: Helix pomatia A hemagglutinin, Soy bean agglutinin, Lima bean lectin, and Dolichos biflorus lectin. *Biochemistry*, 1977, 16, 2750-2755.

[99] Irimura, T; Denda, K; Iida, S; Takeuchi, H; Kato, K. Diverse glycosylation of MUC1 and MUC2: potential significance in tumor immunity. *J. Biochem.*, 1999, 126, 975-985.

[100] Rye, PD; Fodstad, O; Emilsen, E; Bryne, M. Invasion potential and N-acetylgalactosamine expression in a human melanoma model. *Int. J. Cancer*, 1998, 75, 609-614.

[101] Okuyama, T; Maehara, Y; Kakeji, Y; Tsuijitani, S; Korenaga, D; Sugimachi, K. Interrelation between tumor-associated cell surface glycoprotein and host immune response in gastric carcinoma patients. *Cancer*, 1998, 82, 1468-1475.

[102] Ye, C; Kiriyama, K; Mitsuoka, C; Kannagi, R; Ito, K; Watanabe, T; Kondo, K; Akiyama, S; Takagi, H. Expression of E-selectin on endothelial cells of small veins in human colorectal cancer. *Int. J. Cancer*, 1995, 61, 455-460.

[103] Tomlinson, J; Wang, JL; Barsky, SH; Lee, MC; Bischoff, J; Nguyen, M. Human colon tumor cells express multiple glycoprotein ligands for E-selectin. *Int. J. Oncol.*, 2000, 16, 347-353.

[104] Ota, M; Takamura, N; Irimura, T. Involvement of cell surface glycans in adhesion of human colon carcinoma cells to liver tissue in a frozen section assay: role of endo-β-galactosidase-sensitive structures. *Cancer Res.*, 2000, 60, 5261-5268.

[105] King, MJ; Chan, A; Roe, R; Warren, BF; Dell, A; Morris, HR; Bartolo,

DC; Durdey, P; Corfield, AP. Two different glycosyltransferase defects that resulted in GalNAc-O-peptide (Tn) expression. *Glycobiology*, 1994, 4, 267-279.

[106] Irimura, T; Nakamori, S; Matsushita, Y; Matsushita, Y; Taniuchi, Y; Todoroki, N; Tsuji, T; Izumi, Y; Kawamura, Y; Hoff, SD; Cleary, KR; et al. Colorectal cancer metastasis determined by carbohydrate-mediated cell adhesion: role of sialyl-LeX antigens. *Semin. Cancer Biol.*, 1993, 4, 319-324.

[107] Bronckart, Y; Nagy, N; Decaestecker, C; Bouckaert, Y; Remmelink, M; Gielen, I; Hittelet, A; Darro, F; Pector, JC; Yeaton, P; Danguy, A; Kiss, R; Salmon, I. Grading dysplasia in colorectal adenomas by means of the quantitative binding pattern determination of Arachis hypogaea, Dolichos biflorus, Amaranthus caudatus, Maackia amurensis, and Sambucus nigra agglutinins. *Hum. Pathol.*, 1999, 30, 1178-1191.

[108] Tollefsen, SE; Kornfeld, R. The B4 lectin from Vicia villosa seeds interacts with N-acetylgalactosamine residues α-linked to serine or threonine residues in cell surface glycoproteins. *J. Biol. Chem.*, 1983, 258, 5172-5176.

[109] Kawaguchi, T; Igarashi, S; Kono, K. Tumor cell adhesiveness and metastasis-its pathological bases. *Biotherapy*, 1993, 7, 1141-1150. (in Japanese).

ACKNOWLEDGMENT

This research was supported by grant-in-aid for cancer research from the Ministry of Education, Science, and Culture of Japan, Ministry of Health, Labor and Welfare of Japan, and Special Coordination Funds of the Science and Technology Agency of the Japanese government. A large part of these studies were performed with coworkers who belonged to the Second Department of Pathology Fukushima Medical University School of Medicine (Professor and Chairman, the late Kyuya Nakamura). I make a grateful acknowledgement for Mrs. Michiko Hoshi, who works in making figures and tables and in preparation of this book.

INDEX

D

E

F

G

H

I

K

L

M

V

W

Y

Z